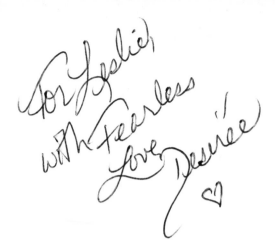

For Leslie,
with Fearless
Love Desiree ♡

What People Are Saying

"There are not enough ways in which I can recommend Desiree's new book *Fearless After Fifty*. Desiree is a teacher of depth, vulnerability, wisdom and soul, and has had a rich life journey filled with wondrous joy and unimaginable heartbreak. What makes her an incredible teacher has been her willingness to do the inner work for her own healing, and the bravery to share what she has learned along the way. Having just turned 50 myself, I am in the process of learning what it is to age in life, and on the mat, and the unique challenges and beauty that come with it. I've known Desiree for years and am grateful to be able to rely on her as a guide on the second half of this journey. I know you will too."

— Seane Corn, Yoga Teacher,
Co-Founder of "Off the Mat into the World"

"Desiree discovered the outer form of yoga through diligence and discipline. She discovered the inner form of yoga for survival due to intense grief. The readers of this book will have the opportunity to discover both as she lays out the magic and practicality of this art form called yoga."

— Colleen Saidman, Yoga Teacher, Director
of Yoga Shanti and Author of *Yoga for Life*

"You could not be in better hands if you are looking to start a yoga practice in midlife, than with these two wonderful

teachers. I've known both Desiree and Michelle for many years, and it's a pleasure to grow older and better with them."
— **Amy Ippoliti, Yoga Teacher and Author of**
The Art and Business of Teaching Yoga

"Desiree's studentship and commitment to the practice have lighted my path for almost two decades. The book you hold in your hands will help illumine your way to your own fulfilling practice, coming from a strong, sensitive teacher whose greatest wish is to introduce you to a nourishing relationship with your body, mind and spirit. May this book move you to become dearly connected with every aspect of your being as you grow wiser with practice and time."
— **Elena Brower, Yoga Teacher and Author of**
Art of Attention **and** *Practice You*

"'My beloved teacher' is how I introduce Desiree in Chinese. Her grace and elegance in the yoga studio brings wisdom that flows from my body to my heart and back again. She inspires everyone to greater health and joy in life. I'm looking forward to taking her teachings with me for decades to come."
— **Benjamin Finnerty, Yoga Teacher and**
Director of Jayarasa Yoga Kula, Shanghai

"Enthusiasm, dedication, humor, energy, and skill are a few of the words that come to mind when I think of Desiree Rumbaugh and her teaching. With precision and grace she consistently brings students to a new level of practice and personal realization. Her deep well of compassion and understanding are transmitted not only with her words but also by her example. *Fearless After Fifty* is a gem of wisdom earned from a lifetime of exploring what it means to truly grieve, truly love, and to be authentically and fully human. May we celebrate life through all it presents. Enjoy!"

— **Bruce Bowditch, Yoga Teacher and Author of**
***The Yoga Practice Guide* series**

"Desiree Rumbaugh is a force of nature! Her joy and enthusiasm for life is infectious. From her lived humanity, which includes the deepest suffering—the tragic loss of her son, Brandon—her spirit soars courageously like a phoenix rising up out of the ashes. Desiree is the shining model of fearlessness who has found her purpose and demonstrates the power of hope and the resiliency of the heart to love and live again. This book overflows with wisdom and insight that we all need to hear. Bravo! *Fearless After Fifty* is an accurate, honest, and much needed look at the realities of yoga and aging. The truth is, no matter how fit you are in your twenties and thirties, once you reach your fifties the 'doorbell' of grace rings. Little aches, pains, and limitations become a daily experience. What I love about this book is the positive, uplifting message that it's not game over, rather, it's game on! Very inspiring and filled with insight, this book is a must read!"

— **Todd Norian, Founder of Ashaya Yoga®,**
www.ashayayoga.com

"*Fearless After Fifty* will benefit seekers of all ages and will give you inspiration to turn grit into gold. It will help you identify and articulate your fears in the spirit of fun, and no better guide than these two women to do that. I've known Desiree for decades and can say without a 'bout of doubt, even the thought of her lightens my mood."

— **Darren Rhodes, Author of Yoga Resource, Model for Penchant for Practice, Founder of YogaHour**

"*Fearless After Fifty* reminds us that the wisdom of aging comes from engaging the worthwhile fights, and letting go of unnecessary battles. Desiree and Michelle know this terrain first hand, having traveled the path through different careers, parenthood, divorce, marriage, death, rebirth and so much more. What you have in your hands may appear to be a book about safe and effective yoga practice, with expert guidance for all levels. However, this is a guidebook for growing older with dignity, to claiming one's own wisdom, and to becoming a warrior for the only fight that really matters—love. Practitioners of all ages will appreciate that this book offers practical tools for reclaiming your right to happiness through the ever challenging life on and off a yoga mat."

— **Christina Sell, Director, San Marcos School of Yoga, Author of *Yoga from the Inside Out* and *My Body Is a Temple***

"In their excellent book, *Fearless After Fifty*, authors Desiree Rumbaugh and Michelle Marchildon exhort us to live courageously, accept inevitable change, and stay strong into our midlife and elder years. Yoga practice and philosophy is presented in a down-to-earth tone, inviting beginners and experienced yogis alike to start wherever they are, building inner and outer strength and confidence. I will recommend this book to all my students as a valuable companion in their life."

"Love lifts us to great heights and throws us into the deepest chasms. Now that I am a father of two small children, I realize more than ever what a precious and precarious balance this life is. Knowing Desiree as she went through the tragic loss of her son, and how she continues to process the pain and grief and love, I have witnessed her persevering strength, irrepressible resilience and courageous vulnerability. Desiree is a true heroine of the Wisdom Warrior path and is a constant source of inspiration to me and many, many others. May Desiree be a light for you to find your own light, even in the darkest of times. Burn brightly."

"Desiree Rumbaugh is one of those rare teachers that present yoga in an accessible, joyful and engaging way. Michelle is unapologetically honest and relatable in illuminating the ups and downs of life. Joining forces, these two women offer their wisdom of cultivating a sensible approach to yoga. This book will surely leave you inspired to practice from an informed and clear way for years to come."

"Show me someone in the second half of life who is continuing to challenge themselves to learn, grow, and change, and I'll see a true yoga practitioner. *Fearless After Fifty* gives students that are 50 and beyond the perfect resource to stay physically, emotionally, and mentally engaged with the yoga practice."

— **Jason Crandell, Yoga Teacher, San Francisco**

"We all crave new life lessons taught from the truth of experience. We want to build our self-respect. Our culture has few guidelines for us, leaving us bereft of a fascinating future. Desiree and Michelle created a guidebook for you, dear Reader, to get off the road to rot and create a life path that makes use of your experiences, thus becoming seasoned Wisdom Keepers. I recommend you read and act on these good teachings."

— **Ana Tiger Forrest, Medicine Woman, Creatrix of Forrest Yoga, Author of *Fierce Medicine***

FEARLESS AFTER FIFTY

How to Thrive with Grace, Grit and Yoga

FEARLESS
AFTER
FIFTY

How to Thrive with Grace, Grit and Yoga

Desiree Rumbaugh
Creator of the Yoga to the Rescue DVD series
and the
Fearless Foodie cookbook

and

Michelle Marchildon, The Yogi Muse
Author of *Finding More on the Mat: How I Grew Better,
Wiser and Stronger with Yoga*
and
Theme Weaver: Connect the Power of Inspiration to Teaching Yoga

Fearless After Fifty: How to Thrive with Grace, Grit and Yoga
by Desiree Rumbaugh and Michelle Berman Marchildon

Published by

Wildhorse Ventures LLC
A Denver, Colorado company committed to producing real voices
in yoga and protecting the rights and sanctuaries of animals worldwide.

ISBN: 978-0-9848755-4-2
Library of Congress Control Number: 2017904042

Editing: Rabia Tredeau
Cover and Interior Design: Nick Zelinger, www.NZGraphics.com
The Book Shepherd: Judith Briles

10 9 8 7 6 5 4 3 2

1. Health   2. Fitness   3. Yoga   4. Body, Mind, Spirit

First Edition

Printed in the United States

Dedications

For all the pain that humbles me, and the joy that delights me in this lifetime. And for my granddaughter, Kyla, who gives me an extra incentive to stay strong and flexible.
~ Desiree Rumbaugh

For the teachers who started me on this path late in life. In fact, there is no such thing as late; there is only life. And for my yoga tribe in Denver. I couldn't ask for better company.
~ Michelle Marchildon

Acknowledgments

From Desiree:

I am grateful to my very creative mother for teaching me to believe in myself. Because of her, I grew up to be confident without fear of public speaking. I am grateful to my super steady father, who supported my desire to be a dance major in college. Who knew this would lead to a yoga career? I thank my children for giving me the great gift of motherhood, which taught me how to love unconditionally. And to my husband, Andrew, who helped to heal my heart, taught me how to be physically stronger, and to play like a kid again. Lastly, much love and gratitude to Michelle, who helped me put to paper the words and thoughts that have been in my heart for 25 years.

From Michelle:

I am deeply grateful to my husband, Mike, who believes in me even when I doubt myself. Sam and Teddy, thank you for choosing me as your mommy. You have both taught me the meaning of love. I am indebted to my yogis in Denver, who laugh at all my corny jokes and show up year after year to practice our way to enlightenment. I would not be a yogi today without Desiree, who taught me yoga with alignment, integrity and strength. I have so many teachers that it would be impossible to name them all, but I would be remiss if I did not mention Christina Sell for her remarkable wit, insight and intelligence, and Amy Ippoliti, who unlocked my fearless heart.

From Both of Us:

We want to thank Stephanie Tade for seeing the light in this project. Rabia Tredeau, or "Rabs" you are truly "Fabs." Thank you for being an excellent editor and yogi. Nicky "Z," or Nick Zelinger, thank you for the beautiful layout and design. Judith Briles, what can we say? We would not do a book without you. A deep breath of appreciation to Jamie Kent and Jackie Casal of *YogaDownload*, who arranged to host the online videos that show how to practice yoga the *Fearless After Fifty* way. Most of all, a huge debt of gratitude to the *Om-Mazing* Cyndi Lee, as your presence in this book, and your mentorship in life and yoga, is a blessing to us all. From the both of us, we are deeply, truly thankful to everyone who supported us, to the Universe, and to our loved ones who put up with us for this project. Namaste.

Contents

Foreword
A Good Recipe for Now

This book is so inspiring that after just reading the introduction I felt like rolling out my mat and doing yoga, even though I was sitting in a coffee shop. I had the urge in part because I thought this was a yoga book. That's understandable. Yoga is the reason I know Desiree and Michelle.

Desiree and I had a passing acquaintance for many years, orbiting around each other within our mutual professional universe. But about five years ago, we found ourselves working together on a project and that's when she told me about a new class she'd been teaching called Wisdom Warriors™, a yoga class designed especially for over-50 yogis. Desiree was not talking about a gentle yoga class for out-of-shape middle-aged folks who had recently awakened to the fact that moving their bodies would dramatically enhance the quality of their lives. Her Wisdom Warrior students were practicing yogis who happened to be over 50 and wanted to engage in a fierce and safe, smart and joyful approach to asana that would enable them to continue practicing yoga for the rest of their lives. That sounded familiar—I was also a long-time practicing yogini and several years past 50. I wanted to meet these warriors and be part of this thing, so I invited Desiree to join me in co-teaching an all-day seminar at an upcoming Yoga Journal conference. We used her title, Wisdom Warriors, and split the day in two, each teaching half of the seminar. It was not only a sell-out event, but we started joking that we should require ID for admittance because there were actually several people under 50 who tried to sneak into the class.

Among the many traditions of yoga that have been imported and integrated into our western world, the honoring of elders has not quite made the transition to our culture. Many people's ideas of yoga come from their Instagram feed picturing mostly young, and wildly energetic yogis, and over the past decade, yoga conferences offering master seminars have morphed into yoga/music/fun festivals featuring acrobatic yoga demonstrations held during organic cocktail happy hour.

So when we discovered that younger yogis were trying to get in on the action of the older, fierce, fit and vibrant yogis, it spoke volumes. Since I was over 50 and so was Desiree, we allowed ourselves to take each other's portion of the workshop. Desiree started by sitting on the edge of the stage and inviting questions, concerns, requests, such as: "Can you help me get up into a handstand?" And, "I don't want to stop doing big backbends, but my shoulder is starting to feel tweaky."

These questions reflected an important passage; the kind of thing that comes more than once in life, if we are fortunate enough to live long enough: teenage-dom, becoming an adult, empty nest, menopause, moving into retirement life. All these liminal phases in life bring identity crises, small or not so small, when we understand that we are no longer the same as we used to be, yet we don't exactly know how to be with ourselves as we are right now. For these over-50 yogis to be able to receive guidance from an expert who was also in their own age-cohort was a huge gift! Desiree's practical and confident teachings offered clarity for their confusion, confidence for their instability, and encouragement for their vibrant mojo.

After the class, as we downloaded our experience with each other, Des said, "I'm kind of like a gym teacher." And I knew what she meant. In the best way of all teachers, she is not so wedded to yoga that she doesn't recognize the value of other approaches to working with one's body. In Buddhism, this is called 'skillful means" and is one of the most important things to keep in mind when trying to accomplish one's goals.

Desiree's goal is to help people over 50 continue having a friendly and functional relationship with their body. To this end, she suggested to the students who wanted to go up into handstand that they do push-ups. She didn't treat them like fragile beings. She made them sweat. She drew on her knowledge of yoga therapy to teach them how to keep their shoulders safe while practicing backbends. Since it's so important to keep aging spines fluid and strong, she gathered everyone into a circle and demonstrated this work with one person at a time. This gave the Wisdom Warriors confidence that they could do so much more than they thought they could and they were thrilled! Maybe Desiree is like a gym teacher, but the more important point is that she is a teacher; one who truly knows how to teach with authenticity and authority. I don't think I'm the only person who knows her who thinks, "I'll have what she's having."

Co-author and fellow yogini, Michelle, has written a book that shows and tells us exactly what that specialness is. She has broken it down so we can taste all the ingredients and then she gives us the recipe so we can get there ourselves.

Michelle is also a master of skillful means, including that of sharing her own transformation story. She started out as a grumpster and ended up living a life of positivity and potential. She did it by being able to really hear the subtext of Desiree's teaching, which is that everything is workable. *Fearless After Fifty* tells us that whatever obstacles we have can be overcome, if only we are willing to accept that we have obstacles, that obstacles are impermanent and that if you are over 50, the time is now. *Fearless After Fifty* shows us how to successfully mix the required ingredients—equal parts heart and mind, body and attitude—in order to walk the path of being fearless after 50.

That is the key. No matter how many recipes you get, you still have to make the bread yourself. We have to walk this path on our own. What is the motivation? Not to feel better later because when you are over fifty, you don't want to think about later. You are all about now.

Being about now *is* being fearless, especially when you are over 50. It's also wisdom, the wisdom of the warrior.

~ Cyndi Lee, Lynchburg, Virginia

But First: A Word About the Yoga ...

We know that some of you have never stepped on a mat in your life. We also know that some of you have been practicing yoga for a lifetime. Here is the thing about the practice: Yoga meets you where you are.

In midlife, our practice supports us. It can be humbling. It can be thrilling. Yet if there is one thing we have learned, it is this: We no longer work to get a pose. We make the pose work for us.

Keeping that in mind, we have done our best in this book to describe how to practice yoga on a sliding scale from grace to grit. But *Fearless After Fifty* is not just a practice book. It is a life book. On these pages, we hope to inspire you to try our strong, engaged approach to the practice of yoga.

So here is the caveat: It is nearly impossible to learn yoga from a book! For centuries the practice was taught through an ongoing relationship between teacher and student. You would grow up and grow old together.

You most likely will need to see a pose to understand it. Therefore, for each yoga pose, or *asana*, we are providing quick and easy video tutorials. They say a picture is worth a thousand words. We're creating these videos to *save* a thousand words and help you on your way.

Videos for *Fearless After Fifty* can be found at
www.YogaDownload.com

Introduction
Can We Be Fearless?

The inspiration for this book came some time ago when Michelle and Desiree each turned 50 and discovered that life was now very different both on and off the mat. Michelle, as the "Yogi Muse," wrote a blog called, *Fifty Things to Love about Being 50!* Desiree created the Wisdom Warriors yoga class and training format with the intention of keeping her students safe, strong and most importantly, vibrant.

So we thought, let's write about how much there is to love about this time in our lives!

If we're honest though, it's hard to love getting older. The changes that occur in mind, body and spirit can be daunting, giving rise to our deepest fears. We want you to know that fear happens, but it doesn't have to hold us back.

Yoga is a worldwide phenomenon encompassing all ages, but in the West it is often culturally represented by youth and youthfulness. While the media is starting to recognize yogis with color and yogis with curves, our culture is slower to embrace yogis with wrinkles. It's as if once you hit a certain age, you need to move over and get out of the way.

Instead, *Fearless After Fifty* wants to celebrate the midlife warrior. We want to encourage you to practice whether you are 50, or will get here someday. If you are older and wiser than us, we youngsters bow to your knowledge. We want our 70s, 80s and 90s to be as dynamic as we are now—or more so! Our most profound revelation is that we are in this together—all generations—to discover how to live the best life possible.

Up to now, the model for midlife has typically been to take it easy. We have been told by physicians, physical therapists, and sports trainers that if your bones are achy, rest. If you cannot sit upright, then recline. If you cannot engage in your favorite activities, then it's time to take up knitting.

We believe that advice is misguided. It was probably recommended out of fear of injuring our older bodies rather than having faith in our inherent capabilities. A host of older athletes today are proving there are rewarding years ahead. This is the time when we must work harder, stronger and smarter to maintain muscle and increase endurance.

Yoga could be an end game for you because the thrill of finding new skills on the mat answers your need for adventure in life. Perhaps yoga could keep you ready for the activities you love, such as walking, tennis, biking or just living pain-free. Or maybe the philosophical tenets feed your inner spirit animal. Either way, we are with you in the midlife trenches.

We know that staying strong and flexible is possible. We practice with verve and vigor, which keeps us steady and our spirit alive. When the body starts to sag, it's great to have at least one thing that does not need more elastic support—the spirit!

Don't get us wrong. We are not in the hunt to stay young or be anything other than what we are. We are not running away from aging. Rather, we are embracing this time in our lives and seeking ways to thrive with our current physical challenges. It is our belief that we are held back by fear and not by our actual capabilities when it comes to pushing our limits. We want you to know there are many things that are stronger than fear: love, passion, perseverance, faith, trust, and even just the grit it takes to hang in there. Grit is not given; it is earned.

You can start now to build a better future. No effort is ever wasted. Even if the body slows, it is an opportunity to let the mind and spirit soar. With practice and a shift in outlook, you can embrace changes and cultivate a kind of fearlessness about life.

Fearless After Fifty also draws from our personal story of how we, the authors, have survived life with grace and grit. You will be inspired by Desiree, who lost her son in a tragic, unsolved murder. She fought hard to feel deserving of happiness again. Her narrative will encourage and support you as you fight your own battles.

Every one of us has a story. Although we can't go back and rewrite the beginning, it's up to us how we write our ending. If we can accept the changes in our body, and work with the fear in our heart, then aging can be a time to explore our expansive and resilient spirit. We all want to live the fullest life possible. We want to walk with swagger. We are determined to live, love, and most importantly, laugh our way to enlightenment.

We are walking each other home, but some of us have a bounce in our step. Be one of those people. We'll show you how.

Lovingly,
Desiree Rumbaugh,
Michelle Marchildon

One
Finding the Okay

Everything you want is on the other side of fear.
~ Jack Canfield

As we approach midlife we have a host of physical issues to sort out that may include cranky joints, weaker bones, mental health, fading acuity, changing hormones, and more.

Then there is the emotional baggage we may be carrying. Relationships don't always thrive. You may have lost some friends along the way. Then there's family. The divorce rate for 55 to 64-year olds has more than doubled since the 1990s, while divorces for the over-65 crowd have tripled.[1] You may even have had to say goodbye to a loved one by now.

If you have made it this far in life and have never had your heart broken, then you simply haven't been doing it right.

This is all to say that it is natural, and even to be expected, that we would become afraid—afraid of losing our capabilities, afraid of love, afraid of loss, afraid of life itself. Fear is our instinctual way of coping with the unknown.

Fear, in fact, has to be the oldest human emotion. We are sure that from the beginning of time there was certainly fear of being eaten by a saber-toothed tiger. Psychologist Erik

---

[1] Susan Brown and I-Fen Lin, *The Gray Divorce Revolution: Rising Divorce Among Middle-aged and Older Adults, 1990-2010*, Kentucky: Bowling Green National Center for Family & Marriage Research, March 2013.

Erikson says that what holds us back from living to our fullest potential is the fear of aging. That's ironic. Fear speeds the very decline in our physical health that we dread the most.

Ultimately, fear robs our life of meaning and becomes our most limiting factor.

But wait. Before you put this book down in despair and give up, this is also true: It doesn't have to be this way. This could be the best time of your life. While we cannot change either our present circumstances or the past, we have total control over how we consider things. We can make friends with our fear, drop our emotional baggage, and begin to live with grace and grit. Everything starts with attitude.

The difference between happy people and unhappy people: Happy people work hard to be that way.

Only one thing separates the happy ones from the herd, and that's the way they choose to consider things. Yes, it's a choice. You are very much in control of how you want to experience life.

"There are two ways to live your life," said Albert Einstein. "One is as though nothing is a miracle. The other is as though everything is a miracle."

We choose the miracle. We want to show you how.

What If You Had No Problems?

Michelle was probably like many of you. She was not a naturally happy-go-lucky person. She is a New Yorker and those from the

Big Apple are not known for their sunny attitudes. They can be grouchy.

Many years ago Desiree asked a question that changed Michelle's life.

"What if you had no problems?"

"What the hell?" Michelle responded.

Until that moment Michelle was defined by her problems. Everything that happened was a headache. She was a "kvetch," which is Yiddish for a whiner. If the sun was shining, Michelle worried about skin cancer. If it was raining, her children would get pneumonia. A good day meant that something bad was coming tomorrow.

Yet problems are relative. You may think you have difficulties until you hear about someone else's life. Then you realize you have it pretty good.

Perspective can put problems in their place. One of our tenets is this: It can always get worse.

Michelle thought her life had been tough—and it had—but then she met Desiree.

Desiree is the embodiment of uplifting spirit and unconditional love. She has an unquenchable thirst for life, a maternal desire to help and heal others, along with an easy, natural laugh. It may seem that she has lived a charmed life, but nothing could be further from the truth. Her passion for choosing to live life fully and for teaching both the art and the science of yoga is fueled by her own experience recovering from deep grief.

It wasn't just kismet that Michelle met Desiree at a time in Michelle's life when she felt particularly low on the happiness scale. It was actually life changing.

Desiree's Story

Desiree has traveled throughout the world for more than 20 years to spread her message that through the steady practice of love, hope and forgiveness you can live a better life. She teaches this through yoga.

To embrace that love is stronger than fear is not easy. Some may say this is crazy talk. But believing in the power of love is Desiree's purpose. She has become a talisman of courage worldwide. To see her standing strong in the face of heartbreak gives us faith that anyone can live a better life. It is truly possible.

Brandon Rumbaugh, 1983 - 2003

Until October 18, 2003, Desiree's life was going according to plan. She was a busy, working mother. She had a yoga studio in Scottsdale, Arizona. Her career as an international yoga teacher was taking off and she spent many weekends traveling to teach a style of yoga that was her unique blend of joyful inspiration and alignment.

Then everything changed.

"On that day in October, I returned to Phoenix from teaching a workshop," she remembers. "I was greeted at the Sky Harbor Airport by my father and two brothers. They told me that my 20-year-old son, Brandon, and his 19-year-old girlfriend, Lisa, had been shot to death while camping overnight. They were sleeping in the back of her mother's pickup truck in Bumble Bee, Arizona, about an hour north of Phoenix. It was their one-year anniversary."

"When they didn't show up for work on Saturday morning, we knew something must be wrong, but they weren't discovered until Sunday because they hadn't told anyone where they were going to celebrate their anniversary. There was no robbery, no apparent motive, and although it was broadcast on national media, the case was never solved."

At 20, Brandon was just starting to come into his own. He was thriving in college and working as a personal trainer, helping people become healthy and fit. (Indeed, the apple doesn't fall far from the tree.)

As a teenager, Brandon was especially creative. He was musically inclined, playing a wide variety of instruments including the tuba, trumpet, trombone, saxophone and guitar. His favorite was the drums, much to the dismay of Desiree's neighborhood. He excelled both in marching band and jazz band in high school, and to this day Desiree's heart swells when she hears the sounds of band practice. He was one of two boys in the high school dance program and they often featured him in hip-hop or jazz numbers. He was also artistic. His mother still has the paintings and sculptures he made in grade school.

Desiree is fortunate to also have a daughter, Jessica, a beautiful and talented young woman, in addition to her lovely granddaughter, Kyla. But nothing compensates for the loss of a child. Nothing.

"This was an unthinkable tragedy. An unimaginable pain," said Desiree. "Losing someone so close and so dear feels like losing a part of oneself. We are never the same; we are permanently shifted."

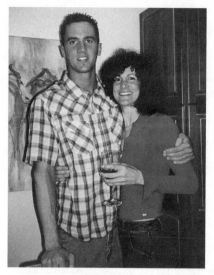

Brandon Rumbaugh at 19, and Desiree

Although she was a practicing yogi, a student of yoga philosophy, with a promising international career, this heartbreaking event marked the true beginning of her transcendent journey. It would have been much easier to stay home, to dissolve in a conundrum of anger and fear, and let life pass her by. But that wasn't her destiny.

"My spiritual journey had begun," she remembers. "My deepest fear at this time was that I would never again know joy. I was afraid that my life would always have a tone of sorrow. So I set out on a mission to reclaim my joy and my reason for living."

After the news of her son's death, Desiree could barely get out of bed. She lost weight and found it hard to face each new day. But in time, though she could not yet eat without sadness, nor walk or talk without tears, she returned to her yoga mat.

"I kept practicing yoga because I thought that maybe by keeping my body alive that it would support my mind. I did yoga by rote, by habit and I was only half aware of what I was doing. My heart was with Brandon and not among the living. Yet after many months, very slowly I started to come back to life for myself and for my daughter."

Little by little Desiree felt stronger. Although she wanted to continue teaching yoga, she wasn't sure she had the strength to travel. Over time she began accepting invitations to visit the studios and friends that she knew throughout the world. As she ventured out, Desiree found herself embraced by thousands of people who loved her and admired her courage to carry on after such a devastating ordeal.

"After thousands of frequent flyer miles and landing into the open hearts of friends and strangers, I realized my son's death did not mean the end of everything. Brandon's passing could renew my own life and purpose," Desiree said.

The Worst Grief

Losing a child is the worst grief imaginable, according to Romeo Vitelli, PhD.[2] "The emotional blow associated with child loss can lead to a wide range of psychological and physiological problems including depression, anxiety, cognitive and physical symptoms linked to stress, marital problems, increased risk for suicide, pain and guilt," Dr. Vitelli wrote. There is even some evidence that the suffering and trauma can lead to a reduced lifespan of the surviving parents. "All of these issues can persist long after the child's death."

---

[2] Romeo Vitelli, PhD, "When a Parent Loses a Child," *Psychology Today*, Feb. 4, 2013.

The work of reclaiming one's life from the grips of depression and sorrow is not easy. Doing so as a result of the death of a child is perhaps the toughest undertaking of all. Desiree shows us it is possible, however. Heartbreak such as this changes us forever. We are not meant to forget our traumas. Yet with dedicated work, paying attention and being determined we can live with the experience, learn and grow from it.

Time alone does not heal all wounds.
But time gives us the tools to endure them.
~ Patti Smith

Though grief still pays Desiree unannounced visits, particularly around holidays and anniversaries, it is less traumatic after almost 15 years. At first, the pain was like a tsunami that knocked her off her feet. Now it's more like waves that occasionally lap at her consciousness.

"I look back and I can see how my feelings in relation to this deep loss have morphed and changed," she describes. "I know from experience that everyone has something they need to forgive, or something they need to rise above. I have often said that if my story can help others, then I am willing to tell it. I have had to relearn and recommit to the idea that love is stronger than fear."

Fighting Back

Desiree didn't have to *find* her way back as much as she had to *fight* her way back. Reclaiming your right to joy starts with believing that you deserve it. Having a life altering experience doesn't automatically make you wiser; it's what you do with it.

Desiree began by studying everything she could about grief and loss. Over time she came to a few significant realizations. The first was after watching *Fierce Grace*, a film by Mickey Lemle, in which Ram Dass, a spiritual teacher and Harvard professor, wrote to an Oregon couple who had lost their young daughter. He suggested to the parents that their daughter had "finished her work on earth."

"I watched that DVD over and over again," Desiree remembers. "I was trying to get my brain to process the wisdom of those profound words."

Today Desiree envisions Brandon's life as being complete at 20 years of age, and that her own work was meant to carry on much longer. She theorizes that in a certain way, a pact was made between them. They were mother and child but only for a short time, and then she was to learn how to live without her child in order to help others do the same thing.

In 2010 Desiree gave a talk at Yoga Journal's Estes Park Conference. It was entitled, "How to Live a Problem-Free Life." Something about this session caught Michelle's attention, so she took a seat at the back of the room.

"What if you had no problems?" Desiree asked.

"What the hell?" Michelle responded.

That was the moment Michelle decided she would no longer be defined by her problems.

There wasn't a dry eye in the house as the audience listened to Desiree's story. Here are the truths she has learned about reclaiming her right to happiness.

Desiree's Hard-Won Lessons on Surviving Hardship

1. Worrying changes nothing. It does not diminish the possibility of events happening, or prevent them from occurring, or alter the outcome. It's a very stressful and inefficient use of your energy. Only you can choose how to spend your time, and where to place your attention.

2. Death is natural, even when tragic. Everyone dies, perhaps not when or the way we would prefer, but it's not up to us. Our anger at life for flowing the way it does is our frustration at being human. We are not in charge.

3. Empowerment is uplifting and inspiring. Being a victim takes more energy than being a warrior. I had to work tirelessly to make sure that the members of my family did not see themselves as victims.

4. We are each separate souls. I came to see my son as a separate soul, not just as "my son." Separate souls are allowed to come and go freely from this planet. It is not up to us to decide how and when they live their lives.

5. Time allowed for healing. People said that it would, and it did.

6. I needed to do the work. There is no substitute. There is no one else who can heal us but ourselves. We are

not stronger because we've had a certain experience. We are stronger because of what we've done with that experience.

7. Value the preciousness of all relationships and life. Take nothing for granted, and know that everything is temporary, no matter how wonderful or awful it might appear to be.

8. Cultivate a deep appreciation for everything, awesome to ordinary. That way you can never be bored or view any activity, even sitting in traffic, as a waste of time.

9. Acknowledge your pain. I honor my son by living my life fully. I know he takes great delight in seeing me thrive.

10. You *must* go on with life. Celebrate joy and participate fully with those who are still living. Holidays, anniversaries and birthdays are especially difficult after a deep loss. I would have preferred never to celebrate another holiday again after losing Brandon. However, if every single person who ever suffered refused to participate in celebrations, our festivities would be pretty small. We owe it to others to live in the moment and not the past.

11. Joy and sorrow are inseparable. Without one you would not have the other.

12. To make a shift, you have to *believe* it is possible. Having faith that I would someday reclaim my life was the heart of my recovery.

13. Be of service. Even when you are hurting, find ways to be useful to others. By serving yogis around the world, they in turn helped me to find my footing again.

14. Cultivate gratitude for everything. Write down the things you are grateful for so you can remember them when times are hard.

15. See life as a choice. There are things you cannot control. Life doesn't always turn out the way you thought it would. Yet you can take responsibility for the portions you own. That's empowering.

16. Adopt a "Witness Consciousness." By shifting your perspective, you may come to understand that things happen, but it's not always about you. You can separate yourself from problems this way, and then make better choices in dealing with them, one step at a time.

Yoga and the Problem-Free Life

The tenets of yoga run deep and across several cultures. The physical, mental and spiritual practices of yoga originated somewhere around the 6th century BCE. The practice began not with the poses you see today, but with a philosophy that was meant to help us thrive spiritually, getting us closer to "a problem-free life." Practicing a pose, or *asana*, was simply a way to help our minds be quiet and our bodies to feel more alive. By working physically and focusing the mind, it would distract us from our emotional problems.

"The body is my temple, and the asanas are my prayers," said B.K.S. Iyengar, showing the importance of the physical practice when creating a peaceful life.

When it comes to pain and suffering, the Buddha would say that to live is to suffer, *dukkha*. But the reason we suffer is because *we attach to our desires*. We think of what we want; we dwell on it; we obsess over it. So suffering exists, but we *don't have to attach to it*.

Buddha would also say that everything is temporary in life. Everything changes constantly. So even suffering is temporary. To be attached to suffering is as inane as being attached to happiness. The end to suffering is non-attachment, *nirodha*. This frees our spirit so we can thrive.

We tell Desiree's story in the hope that it will help others who are suffering from some uncontrollable event of pain and sorrow. Even though we cannot control what happens to us, we can choose our outlook. The tenets of yoga teach us we can choose to attach to our suffering, or not. We can practice the postures without making our happiness about how the *asanas* turn out. With yoga, we have the power to make a deep shift in our attitude and create a better life, even after loss, heartbreak, or sorrow.

"Losing someone we love is a course that no one wants to take, a club that no one wants to join," said Desiree. "But after you do, through no choice of your own, you have the opportunity to gain deeper insights than you ever knew were possible."

Living a problem-free life is about redirecting our perspective. Do we want to define ourselves by our problems? Is that who we want to be? Do we want our entire day—*or life*—to be ruined because of something that happened in the past? Do we want to relive our stories over and over again, stories in fact that were meant to be impermanent occurrences?

Or do we want to use our problems to transcend our situation and make our lives better?

It's really up to us. It's our choice.

A Path to a Problem-Free Life

1. **Get your mind under control.**
   The mind is a problem-making machine, our "meddle-in-law." It attaches to inane things. So the mind needs focus. Get it busy. Keep it concentrated, keep it positive, and help it be quiet with meditation.

2. **Practice non-attachment.**
   You cannot control life, but you can rise above problems with non-attachment. Let go of what doesn't serve. A "Witness Consciousness" means you experience pain, yet it is not *all about you*.

3. **Take responsibility.**
   Own your behavior. Being accountable is empowering.

4. **Shift your attitude.**
   Change your point of view. See life as a miracle and it will be one.

5. **Be grateful.**
   Find something, anything, and savor it. It is a blessing to enjoy each moment we're alive. Victims have problems. Survivors have gratitude.

6. **Serve.**
   There is nothing like being of service to others to elevate our spirit.

7. **Know it can always be worse.**
   Perspective is a practice. Try to see what is okay or good about the present.

8. **Hold the possibility that it will get better.**
   Suffering exists. It is *dukkha*. It is temporary. It is now; it is not forever.

Yoga Is a Problem Solver

Years ago when Desiree was depressed and looking for a way to cope, she found it on her mat. Yoga, she thought, might at least make her body feel good again. And if the body felt good, perhaps her mind would follow. And if her mind would just stop making her life so difficult, perhaps her spirit would rise once again.

She was right.

We live in our bodies. The body is our home, and in the words of B.K.S. Iyengar, "The body is our temple." It is a place for the spirit to rest at night so it may thrive during the day. The body is a shelter for our mind, which can do great things if it is focused. It is our job to keep the body healthy for as long as it is home to our mind and spirit.

However, the aging process, particularly if that includes injury and illness, can make it harder for one's spirit to soar. Emotional trauma is also stored in the body. Very physical aches and pains are often caused by sufferings experienced in the past. It is hard to thrive when you have a pain in your back. Believe us, we've tried.

The Body Needs Love Too

If we have a broken heart, we might think we are doing the right thing by focusing on it. We might spend hours and days reading self-help books, or going to psychologists and trauma therapists. Sometimes that will work, and sometimes not. If you cannot snap your fingers and make your suffering vanish, then perhaps give it a break. Why not? If snapping your fingers hasn't made the pain go away, why not try a different approach? Try focusing on the body. It could potentially be the smallest first step that leads to the greatest journey.

A body not in motion is a body at risk. Yoga teacher Baron Baptiste has said, "Death is coming to a body near you," and that would be the sedentary body. Staying in motion is not just about feeling good; it's about staying alive.

There are two philosophies on what kind of movement is right for us as we age. One approach says that once you are older, you should do less. Take it easy. Be gentle. Don't walk fast or you might trip. A push-up could tear your rotator cuff. For goodness sakes, don't ski with those knees, or ride an upright stationary bike, which could hurt your back. Listening to this advice could make you scared to leave your house! We believe that approach comes from a place of fear. Be careful! You will break! If you do too much, something bad will happen!

What we know for sure is that sometimes you will fail. It's 100 percent true. If you have never fallen, or failed at something, you are clearly not trying hard enough. We can't guarantee that if you get up and get out you won't fail. But we can absolutely guarantee that if you never try, you will never succeed.

If you believe you can live a full and active life after heart-break, or illness, or injury, you probably can. If you believe you can be strong and steady when you feel old and frail, you probably can. You may need to adjust a few things, or move slower, and be a bit more careful, but you do not need to change as much as the status quo wants us to accept.

Nobody should ever quit just because someone else tells them to.

We want to offer you the possibility ...

- *That you are tougher than you think.*
- *You are bigger than what you fear.*
- *You will not break from life's hardships.*
- *What needs to be shaken up is your comfort zone.*
- *You will be stronger if you work stronger.*
- *Curiosity keeps your mind alive.*
- *A sense of adventure keeps the spirit bright.*
- *You are not your story.*
- *You might fail, but it will be all right.*
- *You may not always be jubilant, but you will be okay.*
- *Being okay is sometimes good enough.*

When the Road Gets Tough, You Need to Get Tougher

On your worst days, you do not need to get up out of bed and run a marathon. Absolutely not. On your worst days, you do not need to go to the gym and lift 200 lbs. Surely not. But on your worst days, can you take a breath? Can you notice the inhale, the exhale, and simply the fact that you are alive?

Yoga begins with consciousness. It is from this point that we begin the practice. Inhale. Exhale. Repeat.

As yoga practitioners and teachers, we believe that people only do what they can starting from where they are. On certain days the act of getting up and getting going is a triumph. On the days when we may suffer, it's good to find the okay. We don't always have to be super-duper. From time to time it's good to be satisfactory, tolerable, or just plain acceptable. Without a doubt there are moments or days or weeks when you need to be compassionate with yourself.

The practice of yoga allows for various options of careful and moderate movement. For moderate movement, you can choose: Restorative Yoga, Gentle Flow, Foundational Sessions and Level One groups. There are also Subtle Body Work classes, Hatha Beginning Yoga classes, Pranayama or breath work, Silver Sneakers© classes for older folks and bodywork from physical therapists.

Movement is the most important element in any of those options. Any kind of movement is terrific for the body. It's up to you to know when you need less. And then it's up to you to know when you are ready for more.

We're Old, Not Dead!

Aging all by itself is a journey with challenges. You don't have to have experienced a great trauma to know life's trials. All you have to do is live another day.

As we advance in age, our body changes. And as we can do less, it's natural for the spirit to get a little down.

Michelle was in her forties when she started her yoga practice. In her younger years, she had been a competitive horseback rider in dressage, hunter and jumper events, and even trained racehorses. She also enjoyed skiing and was a bit of a thrill seeker. But by midlife, her back, knees and just about every joint in her body was bringing her down.

"I'm old," she said. "I'm not dead. Everyone wanted me to slow down and I'm not ready for a nursing home just yet."

Michelle is a typical Baby Boomer. We are the most active generation in history. No age group before us ran as many marathons as we do. We love the thrill of adventure! For Michelle, yoga was the answer. Desiree showed her how. "She was the first teacher who looked at me and said, 'You can do more.' It was just what I needed to hear," Michelle remembers.

"Practicing yoga in a strong, deep way is what saved my life," Desiree admits. "The message I received was that once people got to a certain age, they needed to slow down, let go of some poses and reduce the intensity of their practice. Well, I didn't want to slow down just yet. I wanted to practice the way I've always lived my life: to the fullest extent possible. And *possible* is the key word here. Using alignment and skill with the body is what makes the difference between practicing yoga to the fullest extent possible, and just taking foolish risks."

What we know now is that as we regain our strength, we regain our practice. And as we regain our practice, we regain our strength. Strength and flexibility, practice and perseverance, go together like peas and carrots.

We believe when the road gets tough, you need to get tougher. Though it might not be right for everyone, at all times, sometimes you need to discover your potential by working up to your potential. If life knocks you down, you get back up even if it's slowly. That's how Desiree got out of bed those many years ago, and how Michelle found her sassy spirit again. We rise, one step at a time.

Choose to Rise

Life is not always about winning. It is most often about being deeply okay. It is frequently about our staying power and our resilience. There is beauty in simply being here. Steadiness is learned and earned. It's all right if certain days we don't thrive. Sometimes it's enough to find our okay.

"In the end, it will be up to those of us who live with loss to decide how we are going to hold it," Desiree tells us. "We have a choice. We can become victims of life, or we can rise up and accept a new path. I believe that we deserve happiness, even after heartbreak, and that love is stronger than fear."

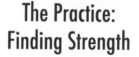

The Practice:
Finding Strength

Begin with the feet

The feet are our foundation in yoga and life. They keep us steady and strong. They keep our poses safe. They support us, so we must support them with exercises to build strength and flexibility.

The core of the foot is the arch, which often needs strengthening. Toes and arches should be massaged and strengthened every day or they can become tight and painful when standing or walking.

Strengthening—Shorten your feet

- To support the arch, "shorten your feet." Stand with feet parallel, draw the ball of the foot toward your heel as if you are trying to make your foot smaller. This will lift and strengthen the arch.

Stretching

- Spread toes by threading fingers through them from the bottom and the top of the foot. You can also put spacers in between the toes. Be gentle. A little goes a long way.

- Practice flexing and pointing your feet. Yoga poses require one or the other, or a combination of the two, called "Flointing."

- Massage feet, especially the toes and arches, to increase circulation. You can use hands or a small ball.

Yoga Poses for Standing Tall

Be strong. Work the muscles in every pose.

Mountain, *Tadasana*

Stand with hands by sides. Shorten your feet. Start by noticing everything: your feet, your legs and your strength. Keep your feet hip width apart, squeeze your short, strong feet toward your midline to wake up the inner thigh muscles. Lift the low belly, then move your inner thighs back until you have a small curve in the bottom of the lumbar spine. Stretch the pose down into your feet and up through the top of the head so you feel taller.

Standing Forward Fold, *Uttanasana*

Keep feet hip width apart, bend the knees and place your hands on your thighs. Lift the arches of your feet and squeeze the legs toward the midline. When the inner thigh muscles activate, push your thighbones back and apart, and slowly lift your sitting bones upward. You will feel a tremendous stretch in your hamstrings. If you can keep your sit bones reaching upward, then keep going into a forward fold touching the ground. If not, bend your knees and start again. Your task is to keep your feet and legs engaged, lift your sitting bones, widen your thighs and maintain a small lumbar curve. If you feel pain, or if your lower back rounds under, bend your knees and start again.

Grace	Pose	Grit
In a chair, work the feet; sit upright with lumbar curve	*Tadasana*	Stand, reach arms upward
Standing, knees bent	*Uttanasana*	Fold forward, with palms on floor

"Easy" poses are not actually "easy."
A video of these poses is available on
www.YogaDownload.com.

Fearless After Fifty: Practical Advice

Easy and inexpensive

- Buy small hand weights and incorporate simple exercises into your day.

- Build awareness by squeezing and engaging the muscles while driving, standing, and sitting.

- While cooking or doing laundry, move up and down on the toes, like a ballet dancer.

More ... money, time and focus

- Join a community or rec center and get trained on the weight machines.

- Seek out a fitness class.

- Buy a weight-training book and study the proper form.

- Groupon, Class Pass and other crowd funders offer affordable ways to try new activities.

- Find a friend and commit to working out with them during the week.

All in!

- Have your body muscle mass professionally measured. Then work to increase it.

- Lift medium to heavy weights three times a week.

- Incorporate Pilates for core strength.

- Hire a personal trainer to learn the proper form.

Two
Keep Calm and Steady On

There is no just.
~ Patricia Walden

We know you want it all. We know you want the chase, the glory, the adrenaline burst of a sweat, doing the things you love, and a job well done. And we want you to have it. But truthfully, as we age we bring some baggage along for the ride. Our bones grow more brittle, and our hearts probably have a certain amount of scar tissue. We might have also developed a few illnesses and other injuries along the way.

We may have temperamental knees or hips. Our fragile necks present new challenges. Who designed this human body, where an 11-pound head is balanced on seven tiny cervical bones? Our shoulders are also open to injury. Instead of being locked in place, the arm is set into the socket by a web of muscles and tendons called the rotator cuff. It's a wonder we stay together at all.

However, we are not less of a person for surviving our bumps and bruises. We are more.

If scars are a roadmap of the physical things we have survived, then the same is true for our spirit. In time we will come to appreciate all that we are, and we'll be stronger for it. However, first we must learn how to live with the changes, and not just ignore them.

So what do we have to do to get that thrill—to live life to the fullest extent possible—without risking more damage? We need to access wisdom, patience, understanding, flexibility, strength and yoga. In time you will see, steady is the new strong.

Wisdom
Definition in Merriam-Webster:

1. *Knowledge that is gained by having many experiences in life.*
2. *The ability to understand things that others cannot understand.*
3. *Knowledge of what is proper, reasonable, good sense, or good judgment.*

What Is Wisdom?

Wisdom is often disguised as patience. We have to be able to sit with what is uncomfortable and then learn from it. It seems that our job is to turn our wounds into wisdom; otherwise they will fester and hinder us for life. Scar tissue is strength tissue.

Many cultures revere their elders. They see strength in years and wisdom in experience. In Greece, for example, one's elders are honored and a severe penalty, possibly even jail time, is imposed for relatives who fail to look after them. In Fiji, nursing homes are very rare; family and friends look after the elders. But before you lament the West as being horrible youth worshippers, know that Nomadic cultures typically leave their elders on the side of the road. So there's that as well! It's good to know it can always get worse.

What Is a Wisdom Warrior?

Desiree Rumbaugh created a yoga training specifically for older and wiser yogis who still want to pursue the thrill of learning new poses and trying new things, and yet be safe in their practice. She works with a physical therapist and representatives of the medical community to make sure she is always up-to-date with the latest research and trends on aging. She calls her approach, the Wisdom Warriors, combining the "wisdom" of getting older, with the "warrior" of toughing it out.

We might once have been thrill seekers and still want that "schwing" in our swing. Or we might now be midlife maniacs who want to keep a sense of adventure in life. We could be entering a stage where we see that the road ahead is going to be quite different than what we have known in the past. We might be wrinkled, but we're still game, and we don't want to take it easy, or rest in a chair, or be placed in a corner. Nobody puts us in the corner!

We still want it all, but the truth is that's difficult to master. And it's especially hard to do it alone.

Even if our bodies start to fail, our spirit and gumption are as active as ever. Wherever Desiree travels, she finds a like-minded community of people who share her spirit and attitude. Whether we are battling aging or injury, we still want to work hard and stay strong. We want to cultivate steadiness. We want to balance on the mat, so when we return to our busy lives we can find balance there, too. We don't want to be put aside or grow irrelevant as we age. We want to be front and center, doing what we can, while being role models for future generations.

What got Desiree out of bed those many years ago wasn't thinking that her life was over. She got out of bed believing that all beings, including herself, deserve happiness. Desiree had to find the courage to rebuild her strength, both physically and spiritually. That is true for any of us who have faced something life-changing.

Wisdom Warriors don't give up. We show up. We work with what we've got at any given time. "It's always something," quips Tonya, a friend of Michelle and longtime Denver yogi. "But if it's not one thing, it's probably two others."

Showing up is the key. Some days it takes absolutely all we've got to get up and go. We, as long time yoga practitioners, know. We're right there with you. On those days your workout is really a work-in. It doesn't matter how hard or how fast you go. It doesn't matter if you succeed at the hardest yoga pose of your life. Often all it takes is one little Down Dog, or a walk outside, or a brief time sitting in quiet meditation, and your whole world is changed for the better.

The enemy, if you will, isn't that you have become older, or that you can't run like you used to. The enemy, or the thing that will cause the most damage over time, is immobility. So on our most terrible, horrible, no good, very bad days, if all you can do is breathe, and maybe move from side to side, and sit up, and perhaps walk a little, then you have won the battle for the day.

Well-being, health and vitality are achieved the hard way, with effort. There are no shortcuts. We wish we could sell you a magic pill, but it hasn't been invented. We have to work hard to stay strong, to get up and get moving. These days, sitting is the biggest problem. A sedentary lifestyle causes lasting damage.

Sitting is the New Smoking

Sitting is more dangerous than smoking.
It kills more people than HIV,
and is more treacherous than parachuting.
We are sitting ourselves to death.
~ Excerpted from Dr. James Levine, Mayo Clinic

Honoring where we are in the moment is wisdom. It is also the key to finding lasting vitality. We can't do things with the stride of our 20-year-old selves anymore. We have to do everything in a way that acknowledges who we are right now. The truth is, some days we will not be at our best. Yet on the days you'd rather stay in bed, those are often the days when your practice is most meaningful. The important aspect isn't how well you do a pose, it's that you simply show up and try.

Nike tells us to just do it. As if that's all it takes to stay healthy, to stay strong, to be steady in life. Just do it?

"There is no 'just,'" commented the indefatigable Iyengar Yoga teacher Patricia Walden in one of her workshops. Nothing is easy. Yet we commit. We try. Sometimes we fail. And then we try again. One doesn't "just" decide to live a healthier life. One doesn't "just" exercise and eat right. One doesn't "just" decide to choose happiness. One doesn't "just" go upside down. One doesn't "just" try again and again. We have to commit. We have to persevere. Exercise feels great when we are strong, but when we are weak, instead of working out, we must work in. Steady is the new strong.

We Got Grit

The truth is we cannot possibly be as strong in our 50s and 60s as we were in our 20s. But here is the surprise: We have more endurance. We are mentally tougher. We appreciate things so much more when they are harder to come by. A child may jump into a handstand and think nothing of it. When a midlife warrior goes upside down, we know the deepest meaning of gratitude. Depending on your beliefs, we may praise God, Buddha, Mother Mary or the Universe! But praise we do!

You don't even have to go upside down to know this feeling of thankfulness. For someone who has lost mobility in his shoulder, simply standing up straight again is a pleasure. For a person with a broken neck, being able to dance in Zumba class may be a gift. We want you to have it all, and return to the activities you love. And when it's time to say goodbye to something that no longer serves you, we want it to be on your terms.

While a younger person may have stamina, we have something much more important: resilience. We got grit. We are still here, and that's not always easy to come by. We value simply showing up in life.

"Endurance is not a young person's game," explains Diana Nyad, the Olympic Gold Medal swimmer who continued to swim competitively well into her 60s. "I thought I'd even be better at 60 than I was at 30. You have a body that's almost as strong, but you have a much better mind."

What Does It Take to Keep Calm and Steady On?

First and foremost, know that you are a survivor. We don't back down from a challenge. We aren't accepting less; we are finding more.

"Since turning 50, we're aware that life is short and the body is fragile," describes Desiree. "Yet we do everything in our power to stay strong in body, mind and spirit. Therefore, our approach to yoga is one of curiosity and a desire to stay active."

Yoga is a path of discovery. The person who stops learning, stops growing. To age fearlessly is to try many things, not caring if we fail. After all, we've probably failed before. What's the big deal? We may fall short of our goal again, or we may succeed. We try not to be afraid of getting a little bump on the noggin', within reason, although a broken hip is a deal breaker. But a little scrape is part of life. We know that if we get hurt, it's a teaching lesson. Next time we might try and succeed!

"I don't even know what 'aging gracefully' means," Michelle said. "Does that mean we are supposed to look pretty? Or does it mean our hair is a mess, we're glowing from sweat and exhilaration, and we get up after we fall down?"

B.K.S. Iyengar once said there are 99 ways to use a chair in yoga, and none of them involve sitting on it. He lived to be 95, standing on his head nearly every day of his life.

We don't want to go gently into that good night; we want to go dancing and diving, skiing and hiking. We want to live our best lives, for all of our lives, and for the people we love. We want to maintain the activities we enjoy, thriving in our physical, mental and spiritual aspects. And when it's time to give up something that may no longer serve us, it will be on our terms.

Yoga is truly a path and a practice that can support us along the way to take us where we're going. Just as using a weight teaches a muscle to grow, we can use yoga to challenge our body to respond with strength and flexibility.

Steadiness Comes With:

- **A buoyant spirit.** Yoga lets us know we are ageless inside.
- **A positive attitude.** We choose our outlook.
- **Grit.** We have resilience. We go onward, steady as we go.
- **Hard work.** It takes discipline to show up, exercise, and eat right.
- **Change.** We adapt to circumstances in life.
- **Authenticity.** People like authentic, original people. Be you and be fabulous.
- **Community**. We thrive with like-minded people.
- **Movement.** We keep going no matter what.

Giving Up Looks Like:

- **Old.** And age has nothing to do with it.
- **A whiner.** Wallowing does not get us anywhere.
- **Clinging to problems**. We live a problem-free life.
- **Attaching to old stories.** We are bigger than the stuff that happens to us. Write a new ending.

- **Stuck.** We try new ways to find a way.
- **A couch potato.** Potatoes grow eyes but they cannot see.
- **Disconnected.** We stay relevant in the world.

Your Body Is Not a Problem

There is one thing that can get better with age; it's our attitude about our physical bodies. We remember our younger days being consumed about whether our body was too big, or too small, too lumpy, or not enough "lumps" in the right places.

However, aging puts things into perspective. It would be crazy to tie our self-esteem to our bodies, because our bodies change at a rate faster than the speed of light! Ultimately, we come to realize that our physical form is not a problem. It's what keeps us on planet Earth. Rather, it is our life's work to keep our body healthy and strong.

"I like to think I am a spirit temporarily inhabiting a body," said Desiree. "My body gives my spirit a home and keeps it warm at night."

"I'm so darn grateful when I get out of bed in the morning and can walk without pain from arthritis," said Michelle. "Aging has turned my focus inside. I've become much more grateful for what my body can do and how it feels, rather than how it looks."

Midlife can bring a certain kind of freedom. The things we spent time agonizing over in our youth may seem silly now. This attitude was coined by Suzanne Braun Levine as the "F-You Fifties." We got the swagger earned from hard knocks. But here's the thing: Don't wait until you are fifty to get that attitude!

"So many young women today seem obsessed with body image issues," Michelle explains. "It takes just one battle with cancer or any serious illness and you will know the path leads inside. The only thing that starts to matter is not how we look, but how we feel."

"We have never met a cancer survivor who was freaked out about her figure," she adds. "Most of us are grateful to be alive."

It seems that with the range of issues that face us as we age, mental health and physical health challenges to name just two, one thing becomes clear: It's an opportunity to focus your attention on what matters to you. If you have waited 50 years to hold yourself in high esteem, perhaps it's time?

Iyengar teacher Cora Wen said that if aging has had one overall effect, it has been to place her attention on what matters. "I feel much more beautiful as an older woman," Cora said. "Old, fat, race, or color, who cares? We need to be focusing on how we feel. If we are healthy and feel good, the rest is window dressing."

If we want to live a problem-free life, then it's time to take care of ourselves. It's time to make our physical health and spiritual practice a priority. It's time to wake up and realize we are beautiful. It's time to value the scars.

It's Half-Time

Midlife is just that, the middle of our lives. It's half-time and we have a chance to strategize how we want to travel the rest of the way.

We know you want to experience that thrill of doing the things you love. Perhaps you used to run marathons or ride racehorses to feel like champions. These days, you might feel like benchwarmers some of the time. The answer to getting off the bench and living fully is in the practice of yoga.

By strengthening and stretching your beautiful body, it can return you to optimal health. You might find that you can once again participate in the activities you love. You might use your yoga practice to maintain your body for playing tennis or running. You might use it to live a pain-free life. Or you might discover that yoga is so much fun that it is just what you were looking for to rediscover your inner wild man (or woman) and feel completely free.

Either way, yoga can get you there.

If Dr. Seuss Was a Yogi

Hello, good morning, today is the day
That you start your life in a totally new way.
With yoga you practice from a bed or a chair.
You do it with company or on a dare.
You can balance on your hands or on your feet.
You can even try it on the street.
Where you are is where you start
You need a body and a lot of heart.
But most important is that you try it today.
We'll help you get started. Namaste.

Yoga provides a light in the aging tunnel. Unlike engaging in regular exercise, where in fact our bodies may run a slower mile, our yoga practice will continue to expand as we mature. We will *always* be able to find awareness on our mats. We will *always* be able to breathe and meditate. We will always be able to find *Savasana*, or "nap" pose. We will *always* have some aspect of yoga that we can practice.

Stay Steady and Strong

Yoga keeps us steady and strong, inside and out, because our body will be strengthened by the postures and maintain its structural integrity. Our spirit grows resilient by the effort of practicing a pose over and over again, achieving incremental milestones. Our mind can become less afraid and more curious with inversions. Practicing presence keeps us sharp.

We also want you to know you do not have to do this alone. We want you to have companionship as we walk, dance, skip, jog, lift weights, do Zumba, climb a mountain, heli-ski, or bike our way home. Join us.

The Practice:
Keep Calm and Steady On

Finding Steadiness

Using muscles in our practice creates strength in our body and steadiness in our life. Older yogis also have older tendons, ligaments and muscle attachments. Practicing with engaged muscles keeps these ligaments safe from tears and strains.

Strengthening

The leg has four sides that need to be balanced in strength and flexibility: the front, back, inner and outer thigh.

- The front: Stand and squeeze your quadriceps muscles to lift up your kneecaps. Build the quads by walking, doing squats, holding a lunge, "wall sits," or seated leg extensions on a chair.

- The back: To tone the hamstrings, stand and press one foot at a time down and back in an isometric motion. You will feel the tone drawing the hamstring and buttocks muscles upward. Repeat this motion in Forward Fold or *Uttanasana*, lying on your back in a Bridge Pose, or sitting in a chair.

- Inner thighs: From standing, shorten your feet. Then squeeze feet toward each other to tone the inner thighs. You can also place hands or a block between the thighs and squeeze inward.

- Outer thigh: From standing, separate your feet to hip distance. Isometrically pull the legs apart or fasten a yoga strap around your thighs and press outward.

Stretching

- The front: To stretch quadriceps, take a Lunge Pose with the back knee on the mat, Hold the back foot with your hand or a strap. This can also be done standing. To increase the stretch, gradually move your thigh backwards and your spine into a backbend. Always keep abdominals toned.

- The back: Bending forward will stretch your hamstrings. Be sure to keep the feet and legs engaged to keep your tendons and attachments safe.

- Inner thighs: Form a wide-legged stance and bend forward. Keep legs and feet engaged as you lunge to the right, keeping the left leg straight, and repeat to the left.

- Outer thighs: Stand with your feet together, then fold forward. Place one foot behind the other, pinky toe to pinky toe, then stretch to the opposite side.

Yoga Poses for Steadiness

Tree Pose, *Vrksasana*
Tree Pose develops balance and requires steady legs. Stand on one leg and lift your opposite foot to the inner thigh of the standing leg.

Warrior One, *Virabhadrasana* I
Warrior One is the first of the standing warrior poses. Stand in Mountain Pose, *Tadasana*, and then step one leg about four feet back. The back foot will point at a 45-degree angle forward. If this hurts, raise the heel to a straight lunge foot and squeeze your feet and shins toward the midline, widening your thighs back and apart. With your hips facing forward-*ish*, raise your arms overhead. Your hips may square in time, or not. Either way, it's okay.

Grace	Pose	Grit
Hold onto a wall	*Vrksasana*	Arms overhead, palms together
Back heel lifted	*Virabhadrasana* I	Arms overhead, palms together heel down, palms together

Be interested in the poses, and they will always be interesting.

To see a video tutorial of these poses, go to *www.YogaDownload.com*

Fearless After Fifty: Practical Advice
Ways to Find and Build Steadiness

Easy and inexpensive

- Showing up is the only thing that counts. So show up!

- Do what you can. If you are injured, think about what you can do and not what you can't.

- Illness means we get creative in finding movement that works.

- Work smarter, not harder.

More ... money, time and focus

- Create a personal reward for showing up.

- Commit to trying a new class or activity a week.

- Find a friend to hold you accountable.

- Attend outreach classes at universities, community colleges, and local hospitals.

All in!

- Set your alarm for new activities.

- Join a club or outdoor group that will keep you accountable.

- Buy a membership to an activity. If you pay, you will probably play.

- Buy a fancy bicycle or spin bike. An investment often makes us follow through.

- Treat a friend where you can share a weekly activity together.

Three
Connection and Community

We are all just walking each other home.
~ Ram Dass

We cannot do this alone.

If you want midlife to be the best life, if you want happiness and health, then you need company along the way.

According to a special report in *Time Magazine* in 2016, "Does Spirituality Make Us Happy?" written by Brian Walsh, the number one determining factor to finding happiness is social support. *Number one!* In order to live our best lives at midlife, we need a friend. Thomas Fuller said, "If you have one true friend, then probably, you have more than your share."

Easier Said Than Done

However, and this is the truth, growing old is isolating. According to a study by the National Institutes of Health,[3] "social disconnectedness" is one of the fastest growing trends for the aging population. This can be either a perceived sense of withdrawal or a lack of social support. It can feel like we don't have any friends, or perhaps only a small network. It can

---

[3] Erin York Cornwell, National Institutes of Health Study on Social Disconnectedness, March 2009, https://www.ncbi.nlm.nih.gov/pmc/articles/PMC2756979.

also manifest as infrequent participation in group activities and outings.

Being socially withdrawn is not just bad for our spirit, it's also bad for our health. The same NIH study found that individuals who felt alone had the identical health risks as those who smoke or are obese. They also suffer higher rates of infection, disease and mortality. This trend tends to affect men more than women, and African Americans more than other minorities, according to Alexis Abramson, PhD, an internationally recognized expert in gerontology.

Despite the amenities and upgrades of our world today, social isolation is increasing. One hundred years ago an older person living alone needed family and friends to help with daily tasks and doctor visits, and neighbors willing to keep them connected to the community. Today, nearly everything can be done online. It no longer takes a village to keep us alive. It only takes a mobile phone, TV and a take-out menu. That can be extremely isolating.

A certain amount of loneliness is unavoidable, however. We may outlive our relatives and closest friends, finding ourselves alone or in a new social circle. Life may take us to a new city or country to be near our offspring. As our mobility is challenged, we may be restricted to activities convenient to where we live. And there will be days where we may not feel well enough to get out and about.

Family ties can also be a challenge. The truth is the longer and better we know certain people, doesn't always mean we like them more. Though we may be related, that doesn't also imply they are an excellent support system, or even healthy for us! We need to choose the individuals we want to spend time with, those who will support us, and who we allow into our inner circle.

Everything and Everyone Happens for a Reason

We believe that when random events occur and people come into our lives, it is for a purpose. There's a saying that there are people who are friends for a reason, some for a season, and some for a lifetime. We say enjoy every moment you can out of a friendship and don't worry about yesterday or tomorrow. Thinking that you will make a friend in kindergarten and keep that friend for life is often like believing every frog is really a prince. In fact, we will have many, many confidants and companions during our lives. Some of them will be there for us at just the right time.

Years ago it was the community in Desiree's yoga life that in fact, saved her life.

"Yoga became my 'Life Support,' physically and emotionally," Desiree explains. "Many of my friends and even certain strangers reached out to share their experiences with the loss of a child, so I knew that I was not alone in my grieving." After the death of her son, depression had taken hold. She could not imagine how her future would unfold. She certainly did not dream that she might one day actually thrive. Her only thought was to survive for her daughter.

It was only little by little that she found the courage to try and rejoin the world.

"Traveling and teaching was easier for me than staying home wallowing in my misery," Desiree tells us. "It was enlivening to be in good company. Though what was really difficult for some time were celebrations of any kind: Thanksgiving, Christmas,

Mother's Day, and especially the birthdays and anniversaries of Brandon's life and death. However, I have learned that there came a time when I had to decide to be alive for the living: for myself, for my daughter, my husband, and friends. During this time, I also felt support to share my grief openly. Many of my students thanked me for being an example of someone not afraid to be real and true to her feelings." In fact, Desiree's courage seemed to rub off on everyone else.

Then something unexpected happened. Although Desiree was the "teacher," it was the community of students who taught *her* what it is to know that love is stronger than fear. It had been a healing mission for Desiree to share what she learned about reclaiming one's right to happiness after a tremendous loss. Now it was her students' turn to heal their teacher.

"Wherever I went, I was welcomed with joy and such sweet compassion. It was the community that ultimately brought me back to life by welcoming what I had to offer."

Community Is Our Salvation

The worldwide yoga community was Desiree's circle that held her and supported her as she came back to life. Each of us may not have an international network of like-minded souls there for us, but we all need a tribe. We need people who "get us," along with individuals who support us on our path. A solo walk will clear the head, but it does not fully nourish the spirit. Our spirit thrives in community.

We are not meant to navigate life's challenges alone. Humans may be the most sophisticated animals on Earth, but we are still primarily animals that prefer to live in a pack. Without a herd, a flock, a horde, a swarm, a community, a tribe, or whatever you want to call it, we are not quite whole.

Being at Home

It was a similar situation for Michelle when she started her family. Like many successful working women, she had a challenging transition from a high profile job to changing diapers.

"One day I was surrounded by like-minded professionals, bringing in multi-million dollar contracts, having my name celebrated in board meetings, and going to power lunches. And the next, I'm covered in spit-up. I wouldn't have changed any of it, not for one second. But it was a very hard adjustment for me."

At first Michelle turned to vodka and Haagen-Dazs, although not at the same time. When that didn't bring happiness, she turned to antidepressants. "I was looking for someone who understood both my joy and my isolation," she confessed. Ultimately, she found community through yoga.

Desiree explains, "Many people do not have the luxury of immediate family or friends close by to rely on for companionship or support. And sometimes our immediate family members are not the most supportive. They may not agree with our philosophy or values in life. I have noticed that with the connections we make through yoga, we can create a community of like-minded people. We can support each other, be there for each other, and at the end of day we can try to age lightheartedly together."

Health and Well-Being

As we said, being healthy and socially active is a chicken and egg situation. Our well-being affects our sense of isolation in that people in poor health tend to withdraw. And reclusiveness and social disconnectedness will have a negative effect on our health. Therefore, taking care of our health—physical, mental and spiritual—has to become our number one priority as we age. If we are full of vigor, fun to be with, engaging and intellectually active, we will be the toast of the party. If we have a positive attitude and a can-do spirit, everyone will want to be with our lively minds and sprightly selves. And then suddenly, we have friends.

"We want to be the relative or friend that everyone wants to have around," said Desiree. "We don't want to be the person they dread to see at the holidays."

For many of us, it may seem strange to put ourselves and our well-being first. It may seem odd to be concerned about our own needs and bring attention to being or becoming happy and content, yet in many ways that is one lesson of aging: We finally deserve our attention. If we have been care-givers for the better part of our lives, then this may be a new concept. Some of us have taken care of children, perhaps grandchildren, maybe also the elders in our family and our friends. But now it's our turn. In fact, we are reordering our priorities to remain healthy for others in our lives who depend on us. You deserve that, and you have to learn to believe it, too.

Isolation Might Be in Your Head

Certain feelings of isolation and separateness that might begin to arise may be just in our mind, since the mind is very complicated. It will often tell us things that aren't true just to watch us spin in circles. Sometimes it's our fear and not our rational mind talking. Maybe we are afraid no one will like us; therefore we stay home. That's when our fear gets the best of us. So it becomes critical that we learn to work with our anxiety rather than let it grow and overcome us.

In *The Work* by Byron Katie, she asks us to question what we think is real. It is a simple but powerful exercise that we highly recommend. Ask yourself, "What if it wasn't true?" Katie challenges us to continually question the world as we see it, trying to get past what we think is real, always wondering, "What if I didn't believe my thoughts? What if it wasn't true?" Remember, the mind isn't always right. Sometimes it's a problem-making machine.

The Malas – Temporary Problems That Seem Very Real

Another explanation for what keeps us isolated comes to us from the Hindu tradition. In Eastern thought, the Malas are problems, not the beads one may wear in a prayer necklace. These particular Malas are the misguided beliefs that keep us from our greatness. They are described as "cloaks" or "veils" that hide the truth. Part of the yoga path of enlightenment is being able to see past these negative Malas.

The Three Malas

- Karma Mala: *Feelings of anxiety, fear, and needing to accomplish extra tasks.*
- Anava Mala: *Feelings of unworthiness, shame, disgrace, sadness, and depression.*
- Mayiya Mala: *Feelings of separation, isolation, conflict, and anger.*

The belief that we are alone and separate from others is *Mayiya Mala*, and it typically preys on those who are going through a change, moving, or isolated. It often targets the aging, the teenager, and the ailing house-bound. It comes into our life like a fog and fills our day-to-day life until we cannot see past our own nose.

Knowing about the *Malas* is the first step to pushing them aside and seeing the world as it is more clearly. In this way, the problems that are the *Malas* can actually become our practice. We can use them to make ourselves stronger. Remember, we advocate that all of us can live a problem-free life. Therefore, we choose to use and even embrace the *Malas* to awaken to our purpose.

Here are a few suggestions: If you feel unworthy or under the influence of *Anava Mala*, try volunteering for a good cause. If you feel hectic, like you can't get everything done, *Karma Mala*, try slowing down. Do less and feel more joy. We promise the world won't stop for one day. And if you feel lonely or abandoned, *Mayiya Mala*, then pick up the phone and call a friend, or take yourself to a yoga class. This is how our problems become our practice instead.

Never Too Late for Therapy

There are three things that continue to grow larger as we age: Our noses (it's true), our feet (yup, still true), and the "bag" we have filled with personal problems. We might be getting older, but we don't necessarily grow better unless we make the effort to change. It's not each experience that makes us wise. It's what we did with it. Further, we need to unload the things that no longer serve us.

If our personality is full of irritating quirks, phobias, and obsessions, those characteristic anomalies grow right along with us as we age. Things that others considered mere annoyances when we were younger will now be full-blown complications standing in the way of our relationships and happiness. We do not grow out of mental illness; we grow into it.

Maybe it's time to unpack our bag? Everyone has a little "crazy," and by that we mean our peculiarities. We may think the things we do are charming. However, the friends and family who have stayed away for several years may think otherwise. If you have never sought counseling or mental health therapy, this might be the right time to explore a bit of self-discovery, and then begin a process of self-nurturing.

Do the work, and it will pay off with new and renewed relationships, along with a sense of well-being. Do the work, stay healthy physically, emotionally and mentally, and our children will be clamoring to spend time with us. Do the work, be the person others want to hang around, and social isolation will be a thing of the past.

Let's Get Physical

It's easy to say, "Just do it," but we know there is no "just." Altering our attitudes, living a problem-free life, staying fit, eating right, and seeking therapy is hard. It takes self-discipline and motivation. Yet here's the good news: It's easier with company.

There are reasons why we tend to pull away from the group activities that were natural when we were younger. Fear holds us back. There may be anxiety that we will get hurt. We're afraid that we can't keep up or that we will look silly.

This is natural. The trick is to accept that those things might happen, and be okay with it. Of course we don't want to get hurt. But we also don't want to live in a bubble. If we allow our fears to get the best of us, the danger is that we will withdraw into our own world. Eventually that leads to loneliness, diminished health, and often depression. We really have no choice but to giddy-up and get out there.

It is so much harder to do this alone. While buying a book on yoga poses or finding exercise videos on the internet is a great start, it is only that: a start. You can't know if you are moving your body effectively, or in alignment safely, if you're doing it alone. There is no personal feedback. Furthermore, there is the huge psychological benefit we receive when we exercise in a group setting.

Group Classes Are a Kind of Therapy

We know exercise will keep us physically healthy, but new evidence suggests that group exercise has mental health benefits as well. Alzheimer's disease is one example. Characterized by a loss of memory and cognitive functioning, Alzheimer's can strike anyone. But scientists have discovered in recent years that individuals who may be at risk have benefited from group activities such as yoga, dance, Pilates, and so on. According to a study in *Frontiers in Aging Neuroscience*,[4] those who harbor a specific variant of a gene known to predispose someone to developing Alzheimer's disease showed real improvement with exercise. Physicians often prescribe group classes to patients, offering a social component to their healing program.

We all can feel the benefits of being with others who share

---

[4] April 23, 2014.

a common goal. Spinning classes are a perfect example of how a group mentality supports exercise. Rather than pedaling alone on a stationary bike, in spinning classes you pedal alongside your "pack." The group keeps you pushing harder and longer than you might do on your own. You might also share a laugh with friends, raising your happy endorphins. That keeps us coming back. Laughter is often the best medicine.

One main reason that we quit on ourselves and on our exercise program is that we become bored, according to the American College of Sports Medicine. One way around that is to get out and join a class. "People stay interested because of the social atmosphere provided by group exercise," wrote Shawn Dolan, PhD, RD, CSSD.[5] "This offers camaraderie and accountability among participants, as well as between participants and instructor."

Whatever it takes, that's what we want to get you going and stay socially connected.

How Yoga Works

Yoga classes help ease social anxiety and the feeling of disconnectedness. It is a chance to realize that we are all in it together. Unlike other types of group exercise where participants are pedaling, or lifting weights, or doing synchronized dance steps, in yoga we often do some variation of the pose together, but in our own way. Not everyone can put their foot behind their head! And believe us when we say, at least some of the time you are probably going to look ridiculous. Perhaps awkward can be the new sexy?

[5] Benefits of Group Exercise," by Shawn Dolan, ACSM, October 2016. http://www.acsm.org/public-information/articles/2016/10/07/benefits-of-group-exercise.

So if you know certain yoga poses will look hilarious, if you know the class will be awkward and kooky, then heck, just have fun! Right? We take the fear out of looking ridiculous because we guarantee that at times you will absolutely *feel* ridiculous. So get over it and get out there. We are all in it together, hopefully laughing our way to enlightenment.

Touch Therapy

Aging well and happy also means we need to have some physical contact with other human beings. Again, according to Alexis Abramson, PhD, humans need "touch therapy," or they should be touched or hugged thirteen times a day by other beings. We need at least twelve hugs a day to maintain spiritual growth; eight will give us maintenance, and four is just enough for survival. However, according to her research, approximately 28% of adults over 55 have not been hugged in six months.

That is tragic.

Luckily in the practice of yoga, we have opportunities for physical contact. There are times when the instructor may touch you to align an arm or a leg into the proper position. Also he or she may encourage partner exercises, which provide a little touch therapy. Of course, if this is not your thing, you just let the teacher know.

Forming a Supportive Community

Now you know the truth: social disconnectedness is a real obstacle in contemporary society. As we age it becomes more of a challenge, causing tangible health concerns. So how do we find community?

There are those among us who have had the same friends since grade school. Perhaps they've continued to grow in the same direction, nourishing and supporting each other. However for many of us that is about as likely to work out as waiting for the Tooth Fairy.

As we age and grow wiser, it is only natural that over time we will find like-minded individuals. We want friends who share our current passions for health and wellness, understand our spiritual goals to be steady and happy, and support our mindset that we don't have problems that we can't overcome. It doesn't have to be an overwhelming prospect to find a new support system. Community is any number more than one. Where two or more like-minded individuals are gathered, there is camaraderie, friendship and empathy.

"I have a studio in my home so I can practice alone and with friends," Michelle said. "With community, I feel supported and stronger."

Begin by finding a group yoga practice where you live. Yoga studios and gyms are often intent on building their community with free events and after-work activities. Many offer social outings outside the studio. Also look for other types of exercise programs that like-minded and similar-aged people are attending. Find a program, join a program, then ask a new friend out for coffee. Just say yes. Explore places that feel comfortable to you. Then you will naturally begin to meet compatible people who will encourage you every step of the way.

Please note that a yoga class is different than a traditional exercise class. There is an emphasis on community connection and support. Competition and comparison are discouraged. If you have never felt accepted in your yoga class, keep looking until you find one that offers an uplifting feeling of kinship.

Technology and Diversity

Adapting to change is one of the ways we are able to stay relevant and connected to the world at large. Like it or not, the internet is here to stay and we can use it to find and form new circles of friends. Facebook and other forms of social media continue to morph into bigger and better means of connection between people. If you decide that you are "too old to learn a new technology," then life will literally pass you by.

We encourage you to stay in the game and keep up with technology, even if you need to take a class to learn how to use your computer and smartphone. No matter how frustrating it is, life only moves forward, never backwards. Don't spend any of your precious time complaining about this reality. Remember, *we don't have problems!* We have another opportunity to find a community class, learn a new skill, and meet new friends.

One of the useful ways to stay relevant and current is to interact with different generations. When we resist this, we can find ourselves stuck in a pattern, same old, same old. We become the grumpy old man shouting, "Those darn kids," or the little old lady who can't use a cell phone.

Desiree points out, "One of the best pieces of advice we have heard is to make sure you always have friends who are twenty years older and twenty years younger than you. The perspective of elders and the helpfulness of youth in keeping up with the times are both critical to our well-being." If you find yourself whining about the "good old days" before computers, then remember those days also encompassed the Great Depression, drought, famine, energy shortages, systemic racism and widespread incidents of prejudice. Do not kid yourself that things were better just because you haven't yet learned how to use the computer.

Every age group has so much to offer each other. Younger people keep us young! They turn us on to new and unique experiences. They show us how to think differently and out of our box. If you don't have young people in your life, then find an activity where you can interact. The same is true for the older generations. They have wisdom aplenty. If you have senior neighbors, friends or family, make a date for lunch or take someone to a museum. Always, when you reach out to connect outside your sphere, the one who grows is you.

Service and School

Service is more than something to do. It is an act of love, and as such, it will bring you more love. Doing something good for other beings actually raises the oxytocin, or happy hormones in your body. When you volunteer at libraries, schools, community rec centers, or animal shelters, you are the one who reaps the benefits.

Through service, we stay connected to others. In yoga, we are taught that we are all here to serve. The trick is to find what we are good at, and how best we can serve to stay relevant and useful in the world.

Going back to school is another way to get connected in your community. Many cities, colleges, and hospitals offer outreach programs and educational opportunities for part-timers.

Online courses are also useful to keep your mind strong and vibrant, yet we advocate that you get out of your house and into the world to take a class. Sign up for programs at your local zoo, art museum, or community college. Many states offer seniors the ability to audit college courses at a greatly reduced rate.

How to Find Your Kind

Another reason to learn to use the internet is because just like Aladdin's Lamp, if you put in your wishes, out pops a like-minded friend. If you are looking for people in midlife who want to stay healthy, active and vibrant, who want to reclaim joy, who want to have that thrill, who want to stay relevant to the world, and who practice yoga, then type that into your search engine, and out will pop "Wisdom Warriors!" Or it will someday soon.

It is absolutely amazing what exists on the internet. For instance, friends of ours recently moved to the other side of the country and were looking for new community. They were older, gay, socially active, and politically-minded. They discovered a group called "Older Lesbians Organizing for Change," or *OLOC.org*. This group described them to a T! Who knew?

When Good Groups Go Bad

Yet let's not kid ourselves; there are challenges to being in a group. Any time you get involved in a collective, no matter the size, you have to work with the individuals involved. The potential for hurt feelings or disagreements arise, perhaps even on a daily basis. There can be power struggles and people who wrangle the group away from its intended purpose. A field in psychology is even dedicated to the study of group dynamics and interpersonal relationships.

As teachers, both Michelle and Desiree have had their share of learning experiences over the years in leading classes and participating in many kinds of group dynamics in yoga. The bottom line is that we are all here to learn and to grow. Even challenging times are often worth the effort because they broaden our perspective and teach us how to be more understanding and forgiving of others. If we cannot play nice with other people, then we are welcome to stay home and have it all our way. The choice is ours.

Making the effort to participate in a group also helps us identify the parts of our personality that may need a little work, or the contents of our "bag." Remember how our problems grow with us? Our quirks and oddities are never more apparent than when we try to get along with others. We hope this is not a surprise, but being lonely is no one else's fault but our own. While it is true that we cannot control what happens in our lives, or the people in it, we can control our response to it. Individuals who have a lot of friends are, in fact, very skillful at being a friend. They have learned how to work in a group and still take care of their individual needs.

Make no mistake, there are times you will find that you must leave a group. Often a group experience will be good until the day when it's not. Additionally, a community-oriented practice such as yoga will have its share of wonderful teachers and classes, and also some that are not a great fit for your personal needs. There may also come a time when you simply grow away from one particular group.

So how would you know if you are participating in a positive, life-enhancing experience or drifting into an unhealthy situation? You may not, but here are some clues:

When You Must Opt Out

- *When the leader does not respect your needs.*
- *When the offering feels wrong for you or your body.*
- *When you have nothing in common with the other members.*
- *If the group does not respect every individual.*

Who hasn't tried something new and then discovered that it wasn't really for them? Don't let a few bad experiences hold you back, though. Be fearless. We both make a point of trying as many new kinds of physical challenges as possible to see what may work for older yogis. Sometimes we find things that are useful; sometimes we find things that are too much. But we still keep experimenting.

Stepping Back: Home Practice, Meditation and Mindfulness

Connection and community will bring you into the fold, develop new friendships, and introduce you to like-minded people. However, there will come a time when it all gets to be too much. Yoga is about seeking the middle path, between community and self, between one's individual needs and the needs of society. You may be having fun at the party, but we need to find a way to be happy at home as well. Home practice, meditation and mindfulness about our community participation keep us on the middle path.

Developing a home practice in yoga is a chance to step back from group classes and make an inquiry into the self. What do you need, now? What can most benefit you? Do you need to strengthen the back? Or do you need to rest the mind? Home practice is where a yogi puts what they've learned in a classroom to use for the self. It's "me" time.

Yoga allows you to rediscover
a sense of wholeness in your life,
where you do not feel like you are constantly
trying to fit broken pieces together.
~ B.K.S. Iyengar

Cyndi Lee, the founder of OM yoga Center in New York City and a respected teacher and author, is a long-time practitioner. When she first relocated to a new state, Cyndi mostly practiced at her home. This has both advantages and disadvantages.

"If a person has never really done very much with their body, and now they've decided to rouse themselves later in life, they will need a teacher," she explains. "They have to figure out their strengths and weaknesses, and then practice the exercises that balance those qualities."

Cyndi said that a first time student cannot really learn how to practice yoga except from a professional teacher. There is too much subtlety in the poses. You need someone to tell you if you are doing it right, and you probably need the community of practitioners to keep your momentum going, Cyndi tells us. But once you are on your way with yoga, then it takes discipline to practice at home. Most of us tend to do the things we enjoy, and leave the hard stuff for another day.

"When I only practice at home," Cyndi explains, "certain parts of my practice can become more out of balance. But when I go to the studio, I can do whatever the instructor asks me to do, and it keeps me in balance." Home practice is the peanut butter to the community's chocolate. Together or apart, each is a delicious treat.

Practicing with others can be motivating, it can be illuminating, and it can be inspiring. A group can encourage us to work a little harder and go a little farther, or deeper into a pose. That kind of accountability makes a big difference and the camaraderie and reassurance is vital.

"A strong sense of community means everything to me," said Cyndi.

We agree. Find your kind. Find new friends. Find company for the long journey ahead.

The Practice: Connection and Community

The Body Is Its Own Community

See your body as a "wholeness" in your life. Begin with the cells and expand outward toward the skeletal, muscular and circulatory systems.

Strengthening

- Shins in, Thighs Out. This action stabilizes the pelvis and legs. Stand with feet hips distance apart. Place your hands on your outer shins. Squeeze your shins to center, while pushing your thighs back and apart.

- Shins Forward, Thighs Back. This action corrects hyperextension in the legs and protects the hamstrings from over-stretching. In a forward bend, press your calves forward, move your thighs back, and lift your sitting bones to straighten the leg.

Stretching

If the hips are tight, then lateral movement travels further down to the knees. It is the job of the hips to open in all four directions, not the knees. Therefore we must keep our hips strong and flexible.

When stretching, keep the feet and legs engaged or you could stress the tendons. You want the stretch directed to your muscles.

- Outer Hips: Half Pigeon variation. From Downward Dog, step one foot to the top of your mat. Lower the back knee to the ground and keep your toes tucked under. As you widen your front sitting bone, keep the foot active and engaged. Squeeze your shins in to move your sitting bones back and apart. Do not overstretch. If you feel a pain in your knee come out of the pose.

- Inner Hips: Stand with legs open to a wide straddle pose. Engage your core and place your hands on the floor or on blocks. Keep the legs engaged, practice "shins in and thighs out," and "shins forward and thighs back" until you feel a stretch in the inner thighs. Always try to lift your sitting bones as you straighten the legs.

Pain

Many of us in midlife will have tears in our cartilage and arthritic damage in our joints. We may be "bone on bone" or in need of a joint replacement. If you are in either of these categories, it is best to consult a doctor. However, giving up or ignoring pain are all ways to make the situation worse. Practicing with patience and persistence will improve your health.

Yoga Poses for Connectedness

See the parts of your body as being part of a community, or a "wholeness" in your life.

Downward Facing Dog, *Adho Mukha Svanasana*

Kneeling on all fours with hands shoulder-width apart, spread your fingers evenly and press your palms, knuckles and finger pads down into the mat. Lengthen the sides of your body toward your ears, then soften the thoracic spine allowing it to descend. This moves the head of the arm bones into the back plane of the body. Now lift your knees off the floor and move the sitting bones upward, working your shins in and thighs back and apart to create a lumbar curve. If your lower back rounds, you are better off keeping the legs bent until you can maintain the proper spine alignment and lumbar curve.

Lunge Pose, *Anjaneyasana*

This is similar to Warrior One, except the back heel is raised. If the back knee is down on the mat, it is called *Anjaneyasana*. From Downward Facing Dog, step one leg forward and place it in between the hands, lowering the back knee to the ground. Keep your feet engaged and squeeze your legs to the midline. Use the inner thigh muscles to move the thighs back and apart. To go deeper, lift your low belly as you extend your spine down through the tailbone, and up through the neck and head.

Half Pigeon, *Eka Pada Rajakapotasana*

This pose will build hip strength and flexibility. From Lunge Pose, place the front foot toward the opposite side of the mat and widen the sitting bones back and apart. Remain engaged in the core, legs and feet during the entire time. Any knee pain will require you to modify or exit the pose immediately.

Grace	Pose	Grit
Tabletop Pose	Downward Facing Dog	Limbs straight, heels on ground
Anjaneyasana	Lunge Pose, back leg lifted	Arms overhead
Supine Figure 4	Half Pigeon, foot at back hip	Hold back foot for quad stretch

**Embrace a sense of wholeness in your body,
and in your life.**
To see a video tutorial of these poses,
go to *www.YogaDownload.com*

Fearless After Fifty: Practical Advice
Ways to Find and Build Community

Easy and inexpensive
- Join Facebook or other social media sites online and look for like-minded individuals.

- Seek out activities at rec centers, religious organizations, and libraries to name a few.

- Volunteer! Inquire at schools, assisted-living centers, zoos, museums, animal shelters, or wherever you have skills you can offer.

- Join a movie club, book club, museum club, or just rent a movie with friends.

More ... money, time and focus
- Try a yoga class, or better yet, try a new class each week.

- Local athletic stores often offer bike, hike and running clubs. Check them out.

- Groupon, Class Pass and other social crowd funders offer affordable ways to try new activities.

- Attend outreach classes at universities, community colleges, and local hospitals.

All in!

- Pursue that degree you always wish you had.

- Join a yoga studio so you can meet people and create a regular habit of attending.

- Book a retreat, cruise or vacation for yoga, meditation, writing, bird watching, or biking.

- Treat a family member to a vacation where you can share a special experience together.

- Host a family reunion and pay for the members who could not otherwise afford to join you.

Four
Faith Is the First Step

People say there are no atheists in foxholes.
A lot of people think this is a good argument
against atheism. Personally, I think it's a
much better argument against foxholes.
~ Kurt Vonnegut

Aging can feel like being in a foxhole. We fend off proverbial bullets from all sides including our changing health, wealth, stamina, and relationships. Maybe Kurt Vonnegut is right. Maybe it's time to get out of the foxhole.

Martin Luther King, Jr., said, "Faith is the first step, even if you cannot see the staircase."

Fearlessness begins with a single step. It begins by saying "Yes, I will try. I want this." Or "I won't stand for that." We have to start where we are, and then we can't give up.

Yet the first step is usually the hardest. How do we proceed when we don't know where to begin? Where does faith and trust fit into the equation of hard work and resilience?

According to the Buddha, there are only two mistakes on the road to truth and enlightenment: one is not starting. The other is to not go far enough.

When Faith Lets Us Down

Desiree thought she did everything "right."

"I came from a very religious background; I was raised Catholic and attended Catholic High School," she explains. "I was a good girl and tried to follow all the rules. But this behavior also set me up for a pretty massive midlife crisis when I turned 40."

It was that year that Desiree's life took a big U-turn. She thought if she followed the rules, she would be rewarded with the great American dream: 2.2 children, a house, husband and a white picket fence. That turned out, however, to be the great American lie. Desiree found herself in a troubled marriage with a person she didn't know: herself. The relationship created when she was just 22 years old fell apart when she discovered who she was and what she wanted.

The decision to break up a family is perhaps among the hardest we may ever have to make. There are no guarantees that it will turn out for the better, or even "okay." This could be our first lesson in faith, when there are no promises.

There are no guarantees.
Where fear is concerned, none are strong enough.
Where love is concerned, none are needed.

Desiree's Catholic faith was shaken, but she had a strong yoga practice and a well-founded understanding of the underlying philosophies, which helped her trust in a new perspective. "Studying yoga and the Eastern religions of

Hinduism and Buddhism for the past 30 years has opened my mind and heart to a broader view of God and the Divine Universal Energy. I have gone from seeing God as a force 'out there' to pray to and ask for help, to God as a power inside me."

"I am still very much a believer in God" she said, "but now the 'God' energy has taken a shape that includes not only a Universal Spirit, but also an individual component whereby I can summon my own divine spark that connects and supports all of us."

Yoga has at its core a practice of "right behaviors" detailed in the Yoga Sutras. These recommendations, including the 10 *Yamas* and *Niyamas* of the "Eight Limbed Path" are meant to ultimately lead to a physical practice of *asana*, and a spiritual practice of devotion. Yoga is meant to unite body, mind and spirit. It is *not* meant to be the belief in a formalized religion. However, it *does* heighten an individual's belief in whatever spirituality or religion they practice.

The foundation of yoga was influenced by the confluence of two world religions that were also forming around the same time: Hinduism and Buddhism.

Hinduism

Hinduism as a multi-deity religion recognizes numerous Gods and Goddesses and thousands of lesser deities who mostly create mayhem wherever they go. Their antics in the stories from Hindu mythology inform our lives the way we use fairy tales today. Ironically, the mythological Gods are not capable of transformation. They are created with one overriding personality trait and they cannot change their destiny.

They blunder along and make mistakes so we mere humans can learn and grow from their experience. We have the gift of free choice, and they do not. We are allowed the luxury of human error and therefore we are the ones who can reap redemption.

The heart of Hinduism is a rich web of folklore and mythology that has grown around the deities, which is thousands of years old. People pray to and worship statues, or *murtis* that may be a photo or likeness of the deities in temples. Most Hindus today keep a sacred table on which artifacts, ancient or new, are worshipped through ritual pujas.

The mythology that surrounds the Hindu Gods provides an underpinning for yoga. Many of the poses include names of these deities. So if you were to practice the pose of the monkey *Hanuman*, per se, then you are practicing to embody his role of service. If you practice the pose named for the elephant boy *Ganesha*, then you are asking for help in removing obstacles in your life. And so forth and so forth.

Buddhism

At the same time that yoga was happening in India, Buddhism was forming in Nepal. Buddhism is quite different from Hinduism in that it puts forth the premise that there is no God.

Wait, what?

It's true. In Buddhism, there is no single, personal "God" figure. There are no lesser deities or Gods and Goddesses running around to create havoc or to save us. There is no Father who art in Heaven who is going to clean up our earthly messes. There isn't a network of priests or holy men. There is only a supreme Universal Energy and Karma that will either reward us or give us our just desserts if we go astray.

Buddhim puts the responsibility for your life and destiny squarely in your lap.

The teachings came from Siddhartha Gautama, the Buddha. As a prince, he was born into a life of wealth and privilege, living in a gated community surrounded by splendor, magnificence and beautiful people.

Then one day, as the story goes, Siddhartha asked to go on a carriage ride outside the pearly gates of his family compound. What he saw stunned him. There were old and sick people. There were starving beggars and lepers. Everywhere he looked, there was hardship and misery.

"Why is that man walking with so much difficulty?" he asked, according to legend.

"Because he is suffering," replied his charioteer.

This was the beginning of the end of Siddhartha, and the rebirth of the man who would be known as the Buddha. The next day Siddhartha, at age 29, left his kingdom, his wife and newborn son, to dedicate the rest of his life to understanding the nature of suffering. In time, the Buddha revealed to his followers the Four Noble Truths.

The Four Noble Truths

- *Suffering Exists* (dukkha).

- *Suffering exists because we attach to our desires* (samudaya).

- *Suffering ceases when attachment to our desires ceases* (nirhodha).

- *Freedom from suffering happens when we practice the Eightfold Path* (magga).

In many ways, our ability to cope with life is our ability to cope with change. And our ability to cope with change goes hand in hand with our ability to endure suffering and discomfort. After all, not everything, always, goes our way. Sorrow, misery, pain and grief are part of the human experience. Misery will not cease to exist no matter how many wishes upon a star we make. Therefore, we have to learn how to be okay when things don't go our way.

If we decided that no matter what happened in our lives, that we would see the "okay," then to suffer would be a choice. For example, there is misfortune, and then there is our attitude about it. Bad things happen, but suffering over it is deliberate.

Some of us may be able to rely on our own inner strength to power through adversity. Others may seek comfort with prayer. There is no one way out of a foxhole; many paths will work. But having faith is the first step.

Faith in something, *anything*, can take many forms. A person can believe in single or multiple deities, a vast Universal Energy, a nice Jewish boy who thought he was the Messiah, or an elderly gentleman with a white beard sitting on a throne in the sky. It is incredibly helpful, no matter what one believes, that one has confidence that somehow, someone, something, somewhere, some energy is conspiring for you. That's all we are saying. Just believe.

"I used to pray to God for help," Desiree tells us. "Now when I hear myself saying 'Dear God, please grant me this' or 'Thank you for this,' I change it to 'Dear Me, thank you!' This has been incredibly empowering in my life."

God Is Everywhere, Even in Bathrooms

Michelle found her religion in a bathroom.

She came from what was once known as a broken family. Her parents divorced when she was three, and at that time her mother began a journey of self-discovery that was unconventional at best. At times they lived on a boat; at times they traveled with a theater troupe. They were living a '60s kind of life of peace, love and experimentation.

Then one day, Michelle's estranged father realized that she had not been going to school! The choice for her mother was either settle down or Michelle would go to a boarding school. Michelle left the next year.

At 12, Michelle had a jaunty little walk that resembled the street smarts of a grown woman. Her adventures with her mother had given her a fearless attitude.

And then she was not.

There was something that made Michelle a target. Perhaps it was the way she held her shoulders back and proud. Perhaps it was because she weighed not more than 100 pounds. Whatever it was, everything changed when the boys found her one Sunday afternoon.

"What have we got here?" the first one said. He was a teenager, and he had three more boys in tow. The rest of the story goes as one would imagine. After the first boy finished, he turned to his crew and said, "Your turn."

All violent attacks are different, but they leave their victims the same: with a profound sense of loss. Michelle lost her light for a while. Her innocence and audacity were taken. A clear before and after existed. She lost trust. Yet this is key, *she did not lose faith*. In fact, if she had been unsure about God before this day, it might have also been the moment when she found Him.

The Moment of Grace

In our lives we each may have a pivotal moment when things become clear. Perhaps when the Universe pulled back a curtain to reveal a particular truth, or we suddenly recognized something that we couldn't see before. Maybe we perceived someone in a new light, or heard something that we innately knew to be true. This was just such a time. When the situation could have become very much worse, it did not. What's more, Michelle knew she was not alone.

Although she was badly injured, which included a broken shoulder, she had one thought: "I am alive." For whatever else would happen that day, and for the rest of her life, Michelle knew she was a survivor.

We are bigger than the stuff that happens to us.

Michelle felt that there was a spirit with her. It was a moment of Grace.

"I knew I was going to live," she said. "I don't know how, or why, but it was as if I could see the end of the story. I knew

I was going to walk out of there and live the rest of my life extremely well."

Somehow, or someone, or something had stopped these other boys. Instead of taking "their turn," they ran away. "I knew then that God was with me."

The God Gene

No matter if you were raised in a strict Catholic environment, or in a bohemian adventure, there is now a documented genetic component that creates in us a tendency to believe, or not to believe, in a man, or woman, or spirit, or unicorn, upstairs.

In 2004 Dean Hamer, PhD, a Harvard educated geneticist, discovered a gene he named VMAT2. This chromosome, along with a pattern of other genetically determined characteristics, predicted a person's likelihood to believe in God. He called it, The God Gene.[6]

Believing in God is separate from whether or not you participate in a formal religion. It is different from celebrating holidays such as Christmas or Easter. You can decorate your house, and hang stockings from the mantel, but in your heart of hearts you will know your own truth. Either you got the gene, or you don't.

"Once I read about The God Gene, so many things began to make sense," Michelle tells us. "I definitely have it. I am 'all in' when it comes to God. In my family, there are individuals who seem to fully believe, and others who are half-hearted when it comes to religion. Now I understand why."

---

[6] Dean H. Hamer, *The God Gene: How Faith is Hardwired into our Genes*, NY: Doubleday, 2004.

There is a broad range of how humans bring hope, faith or courage into their lives, regardless of genetics. The latest scientific evidence shows that the ability to believe, to trust, to feel optimistic about the future, and to have a spiritual component, whether or not you believe in a "God" per se, is one of the key criteria for creating and maintaining happiness.

"When it comes to religion and spirituality, it may not be what you believe or how you believe that protects you from unhappiness, so much as the fact that you believe at all," wrote Bryan Walsh.[7] "And that you practice those beliefs with other people," he said.

The Social Component

From prayer to worship, meditation to contemplation, sharing an individual experience in a group can strengthen our ties to hope and an optimistic point of view.

Deepak Chopra, MD, even recommends group meditation classes that have been shown to reinforce an individual's commitment to self-study. "We all lead busy lives, and even the best intention to meditate can get lost once in a while," he wrote on his website. "Joining a group can make you more committed to your practice. But a group can also represent a meditation lifestyle that inspires every member."

Anne Lamott, a writer who was famously raised atheist and is now a born-again Christian, also advocates the power of group worship. "I go to church every Sunday, which is like going to the gas station once a week and really, really filling up."

---

[7] *Time* Magazine special report, "Does Spirituality Make You Happy?," 2016.

However, going to a church or synagogue is not for everyone. Organized religion can feel dogmatic to those who don't buy in to all the tenets. Further, it feels especially awkward for anyone who does not have The God Gene.

The Minority Experience

Being in the minority is like being the odd one out; everyone should experience it at least once in their lives to understand and be sympathetic to "minority stress." If you find that you are the only Jew in a Christian community, it is stressful. If you are the only person of color in a room full of whites, it is stressful. If you are the only non-believer in church, or non-possessor of The God Gene, it is stressful. If you are the only conservative in a room of liberals, it is stressful. If you think you are the only LGBTQ person in your community, it is stressful. These anxieties can lead to isolation, depression and in certain cases, suicide.

According to the National Institutes of Health, "Minority stress refers to stressors that are related to one's minority status." Such factors can be religious, political, racial/ethnic and sexual preference. Any "differentness" can be a trigger for individuals to experience isolation, stigma and prejudice.[8]

The feeling of separateness is also common in organized religion. Freedom of thought is hardwired into our DNA; it is the very definition of being human. We have the right to think and to choose for ourselves. When a religious community adopts a majority worldview, and you happen to think differently, it can be isolating and disturbing. Instead of filling

---

[8] http://www.ncbi.nlm.nih.gov/pmc/articles/PMC3796016/.

up your spiritual tank, you might feel the life force seeping out of you.

We don't want that! We want to create a society that is based on inclusiveness, where we all rise together. We want to help each other feel comfortable and accepted. We want to support each other, because being in a foxhole of any kind is not healthy.

To take that first step toward inclusiveness, or better health, or meeting new friends, or cultivating a new attitude —whatever we are battling—is huge. It's not really a step. It's more like a leap. So how do you get a little oomph in your spiritual tank if you are feeling out of gas?

Yoga!

If you want that "hallelujah" moment, if you want to find like-minded individuals who are willing to take a leap into the unknown, if you want to feel breathtakingly alive and deeply in touch with the mystery that is life, you don't necessarily have to go to a place of traditional worship (aka organized religion). If you simply want to tap into abundance, believe in the betterment of man, practice fearlessness over fear, increase your trust factor, and find a way out of the foxhole, try the yoga room.

Finding Our Faith

Yoga is not a church or religion. You do not *worship* a deity, even if your instructor might talk about one in class. There is no priest or priestess or shaman, yet some may refer to themselves as such. If this makes you uncomfortable, then go to another studio. You can believe in any religion, or no religion, and you should still feel welcome in a yoga room.

Although yoga is not a religion, *it is meant to cultivate spirituality in each of us.* There is no mistaking the trust factor when we move into an inversion. A certain amount of skill is required; then there is an amount of "let go and let God."

This "God" or Divine Strength is both within and without. Your own inner steadiness and resilience is a powerful energy inside you. This is very important to remember. Yoga shows us we are stronger than we thought, and we have a toughness we can rely on.

Yoga also reveals that there is a certain amount of faith we can cultivate in an aspect of Divine Energy outside of our physical body. It's what is needed to take the first step to get out of the hole. To try a pose we've never seen, to do something unfamiliar, requires a degree of trust in both our inner and outer source of strength.

"I often use the phrase, 'Leave it to the Universe to decide,'" Desiree attests. "I feel a connection to the greater Whole, and I know that I don't have the entire picture; I only have my small view."

If religion is man's attempt to understand the unknown, then part of yoga is to know the mysterious self. Yoga offers a path that has the potential to produce happiness, contentment and enlightenment.

For example, let's look at the sound of "Om," a mantra that is often repeated before or after a class. It has many purposes; one is to recognize the creation and continuation of the Universe. Another is to join voices together in a demonstration of community. Still another is to quiet and soothe the restless mind. Lastly, it is a ritual that like all rituals, whether brushing one's teeth or clicking one's heels, can establish calm and relieve anxiety.

The Mind Is Not a Believer

While you may or may not possess a God Gene, one thing that is definitely not a believer is your mind. No matter how hard you work to cultivate optimism, to believe that everything will work out and trust in things you cannot see, the mind is never going to go along with the program.

Our mind is a foil. It is where the ego lives. The mind is meant to keep us safe. If you decide one day that you can fly without an airplane, and you want to jump off a building, it's the rational mind and ego that says, "No! Don't be ridiculous."

However, if you want to try a handstand, and even if you know what you are doing, the mind will also pipe up and say, "No! Don't be ridiculous." It's a refrain the mind declares when it's confronted with something new. "No! No! No! Don't do it," is the only song it knows! Sometimes you have to invoke a little faith to tell the mind, "Thank you for sharing," or "Shut the heck up," and move on.

The mind is terrified and is a terrible team player. When you try new things, it is the mind, and not the body or the spirit that is ready to quit. When your yoga teacher says, "Let's go upside down," the mind often replies, "time to go to the bathroom."

To be successful at yoga is actually to be able to quiet the mind, and then refocus it. When we succeed in our practice, the mind becomes non-interruptive. In fact, it helps us by being focused in concentration.

Of the mind, body and soul, the mind can be the most irritating. Right when you need support to get outside your comfort zone, it chimes in with the most annoying things. "Don't," the mind scolds. "You are going to get hurt. You are going to look foolish. You are going to be a disaster. You are going to break a leg." No matter what you accomplish, the mind is quick to say, "Be afraid, be very afraid! And by the way those pants make you look terrible!"

To reach our fullest potential, to overcome our fears, we have to find a way to quiet the mind. We need to tap into our ability to doubt our doubts, and believe in the triumph of possibility. "May your choices reflect your hopes and not your fears," said Nelson Mandela.

The Yoga Sutras

Back in the day, the day being around 200-400 BCE,[9] the guidelines for yoga were created by a sage, Sri Patanjali. It was common then for teachings, including sacred texts, to be preserved and transmitted orally. We do not know when or by whom the Yoga Sutras first made the transition to written form. Sri Patanjali is called the "Father of Yoga," but the essential teachings are so ancient that no one knows for certain when they started.[9]

Patanjali's *The Yoga Sutras*, 196 stanzas or aphorisms, are a guide to how and why we practice yoga. Buried in the verses are instructions for how to live life as a yogi called The Eight Limbs. The yoga poses or *asanas* are only one limb of the path, however. The *Yamas* and *Niyamas* are two of the other limbs, which are likened to a yogic Ten Commandments. While Western religions encourage their believers to follow the commandments or else they will be committing sins,

---

[9] Jaganath Carrera, *Inside the Yoga Sutras: A Comprehensive Sourcebook for the Study and Practice of Patanjali's Yoga Sutras*, Buckingham, VA: Integral Yoga Publications, 2006

yogis are encouraged to follow the sutras to promote a peaceful life. It's not about being right or wrong. It's about choosing alignment with the path.

The Eight-Limbed Path

1. *Yamas* – the five universal moral restraints:

- *Ahimsa* – non-violence, non-judgment, not harming

- *Satya* – truthfulness and honesty

- *Asteya* – not stealing

- *Brachmacharya* – virtuous habits, no excesses, and sexual fidelity

- *Aparigraha* – non-hoarding, non-grasping, or non-attachment to possessions

2. *Niyamas* – the five individual self-observances:

- *Sauca* – cleanliness and purity

- *Santosa* – contentment

- *Tapas* – a burning desire for wisdom

- *Svadhyaya* – self-study

- *Isvara Pranidhana* – devotion to a higher power

3. *Asana* – The practice of physical yoga postures

4. *Pranayama* – Control over the breath and the movement of energies

5. *Pratyahara* – Withdrawal of the mind from the domination of the senses

6. *Dharana* – Focused concentration, with an emphasis on belief in universal love

7. *Dhyana* – Meditation

8. *Samadhi* – A feeling of being one with the Universe, often regarded as "enlightenment."

As one can see, the practice of yoga neither excludes nor includes the specific belief in God. There is emphasis on believing in a higher power and universal love, as well as recognizing the divine source of energy within, but the teachings do not specifically mention "God."

If it is helpful to focus the mind on a man in a white robe, then so be it. If it is not helpful, then one can focus the mind on anything else that supports one's practice. Michelle had a teacher who once said, "If you love your car, then focus your mind on it." The object you choose is not as important as the focused concentration, or dharana. The yogi's view is that you cannot live a completely peaceful life until you have a peaceful mind. Therefore, a peaceful mind naturally produces more conscious decisions in one's life.

B.K.S. Iyengar felt that one component of a peaceful mind is to nurture concentration with an emphasis on divinity. In his view, divinity is not necessarily a God outside us, but an energy that controls and shapes the Universe starting from within us. It is the spark inside each of us that makes us great, or indicates our truest potential.

If we clean and tidy our house long enough,
we might notice Divinity has
been sitting in it all along.
~ B.K.S. Iyengar

In *Light on Yoga*, Mr. Iyengar's guidebook for modern day practice, he wrote that to be completely devoid of any belief in a higher energy is to be bereft of a guiding faith. "A ship needs ballast to keep her on an even keel, and the helmsman needs a star to steer her by," he wrote. A person also needs faith in a Universal energy, "to keep his mental equilibrium."

Without a little faith, or belief in magic, or trust in the unknown, someone can become so narcissistic that they believe they are the sole doer, creator and controller of the world. That's a lot of responsibility for one little human! It does not take long on the yoga mat to realize that we are hardly in control of everything that happens. It's often difficult just to regulate our own poses and breath. Yoga is humbling, and it's meant to be that way.

The Buddhist Way

Yoga was born out of the Hindu tradition. However, it was also profoundly influenced by Buddhism, the foundation of which is The Eightfold Path. We summarize it here to give another perspective on how we work with faith without a "God" figure.

Buddha's Eightfold Path[10]

1. Right view or understanding. *(Samma[11] -Ditthi)*

2. Right thought or attitude. Acting from love and a practice of letting go. *(Samma-Sankappa)*

3. Right Speech. Clear, truthful, uplifting and non-harmful communication. *(Samma-Vaca)*

4. Right or Integral Action. *(Samma-Kammanta)*

5. Right Livelihood. Based on ethical action and non-exploitation. *(Samma-Ajiva)*

6. Right Effort and Energy. A focus on healing and wholeness. *(Samma-Vayama)*

7. Right Mindfulness. Developing awareness of all things. *(Samma-Sati)*

8. Fixed, focused concentration. Consciousness, enlightenment (nirvana). *(Samma-Samadhi)*

Many Roads Lead Home

Peace and harmony in our lives is the ultimate goal; it is the way home. One does not need to be a Christian, or a Buddhist, or a thissa, or a thatta, to find peace of mind. Spirituality is simply the concept of inviting something "more" into our world. Religion is another way to make sense of the mysteries of life. Faith is a factor of trust, hope, and divine goodness

---

[10] Adapted from *thebuddha.net*

[11] The Sanskrit word *Samma* can be translated as right, prefect, whole proper, thorough, integral or complete. It does not confer a meaning of right versus wrong.

which we embrace in our everyday existence. It is knowing that we are not the sole doer or controller of the Universe. It is recognizing that we are not in charge, and being mostly okay with that.

It is just as easy to believe that the Universe is conspiring for us, as it is to believe the opposite.

Spirituality and Aging

Developing a spiritual perspective on aging has also been shown to increase our longevity. Research shows that individuals with an active involvement in a church or any type of spiritual community live on average seven years longer than those who don't, according to Lewis Richmond, author of *Aging as a Spiritual Practice*.[12]

And yet, among those age 50 and older, participation in formalized churches is at an all-time low, according to Barna Research.[13]

If this is you, then perhaps try finding your "religion" on a yoga mat.

How Yoga Works

Those of us in midlife today are used to winning. But aging, unlike most events, cannot be conquered. We can't "kick its ass." It can't be "beaten." And that's troublesome for many of

---

[12] Lewis Richmond, *Aging as a Spiritual Practice: A Contemplative Guide to Growing Older and Wiser*. NY: Penguin Group, 2012.

[13] Michelle Van Loon, "The Midlife Church Crisis," *Christianity Today*, Sept. 3, 2014.

us. We have to learn how to live with what we cannot control. That's where faith enters.

Age and time are going to wear away our physical bodies, but we can still have that "hallelujah" moment in our spirit. If you want to believe you can do something impossible, if you want to feel closer to God or just plain alive, if you want to feel that for a second you have been to the mountaintop, then try a handstand! Or perhaps start with Downward Facing Dog. Everyone has a different size mountain to climb.

There are all kinds of yoga that will deliver all kinds of thrills. There are gentle practices for people who cannot walk, or who may be suffering with illness and immobility. For them, a moment of movement is like climbing Mt. Everest. There are practices for anxiety that can cultivate a peaceful mood. And then there are the very physical practices where we stand on our hands or fold into a pretzel. Whatever you are seeking, it can be found on a yoga mat.

"The poses I could do years ago without effort are more meaningful to me now because even though they are harder, they keep me in the game," said Desiree. "Even if they aren't as beautiful on the outside, or if they take twice as long, I feel much more beautiful and powerful on the inside when I practice them."

For Michelle, the part of the practice that keeps her young are inversions. "I never did a handstand when I was young," she admits. "I wasn't a gymnast or a ballerina or even coordinated. So to do these things now is a thrill."

We urge you to try something "impossible." We want you to feel slightly ridiculous. We hope you never give up. We want to inspire you to think way outside the box of what you can imagine, and take a giant leap of trust in the Universe.

Of course you need to learn how. You will need to consider the limits of your capabilities and your level of physical fitness. You will want to learn the technique and the skills to keep you safe. But you also want to throw a little caution to the wind and jump in. Trust more and fear less.

Age by itself is not a factor in how old you feel. You are never too old to try. You are never too cynical to have some faith. You are never too sane to employ a little magical thinking that will carry you above and beyond your dreams. It is never too late to get out of a foxhole. Ask for help, believe in hope, do the work, and trust in your inner strength.

As Hunter S. Thompson put it, "Call on God, but row *away* from the rocks."

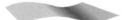

The Practice: Finding Faith

Faith Begins with a Strong Core

Your core muscles literally keep you together under pressure. They also keep your back pain-free. Having a strong core is like adding a little insurance to your faith when you go upside down.

Strengthening

- **Abdominal Bracing**

  Lie on your back, feet on the floor, and place a strap under the part of your back that lifts the highest from the ground. Press down with your core onto the strap and see if you can create enough strength to hold the strap steady while gently tugging at it. Do not let it move. If you can pull it out, then you need to increase the "corset" or the effect of a rib anchor. You don't have to press your back flat, or tuck your pelvis in this exercise. Simply work on strengthening your corset.

- **String of Pearls**
  Sit with your legs outstretched in front. Flex your feet and engage your leg muscles. With arms extended in front, gradually lower yourself to the floor one vertebrae, or pearl, at a time. If this is too difficult, wrap a yoga belt around your feet and holding it with the hands, use it to lower yourself carefully.

- **Half Boat,** *Ardha Navasana*
  Lying on your back, bend legs to a ninety degree angle and hold the backs of your thighs. Slowly lift your head and shoulders off the floor and work to knit your abdominals together. This action glues the chest and pelvis together and builds your rib anchor. Holding this strength, extend one or both legs forward close to the floor. Keep the feet engaged or flointed.

Stretching
- **Cat and Cow.** In a Tabletop position with hands and knees on the ground, slowly lift and lower your head and tail like a Halloween cat and a cow. Begin with your tailbone and similar to a string of pearls, move gradually to articulate each one of your "pearls" or spinal vertebrae. Notice if any seem stuck.

Inversions

- All the principles of the feet and legs apply in inversions, with the addition of a strong core. Forearm stands and handstands are beneficial beginning inversions. Practice inversions by a wall until you are steady so as not to risk serious injury by a fall.

Arm Balances

- Arm Balances such as Crow can be either fun or frustrating, you choose. Mostly they are a matter of architecture, core strength and gumption. Be sure to lean into the pose and use your core to balance. A pile of blocks, bolsters, blankets or pillows makes for a soft landing. Start by lifting just one foot at a time, and keep going until you feel weightless in the posture.

Yoga Poses for Strength and Faith

Inversions are baby steps to bravery.
The core keeps us together.

Boat Pose, Full *Navasana*

Lie on your back, bend your knees and hold on to the backs of your thighs. Engage your entire body, use your strong core and lift your shoulder blades off the floor rounding the upper back. Stretch your arms and legs as you rise up in a V shape. Breathe steadily and stretch through your legs and feet as well as up through the back of your head.

Handstand, *Adho Mukha Vrksasana*
and Forearm Stand, *Pincha Mayurasana*

For Handstand, begin in Downward Facing Dog, facing a wall, press your hands down firmly. Lengthen the sides of your body and allow your thoracic spine to descend. Keep your "corset" strong as you take a step in with one foot. Lift the back leg, keeping it straight. As you kick up to the wall, keep your arms and legs as straight as possible. Forearm Stand is similar in that you press down on your forearms and wrists instead of your hands.

Crow Pose, *Bakasana*

Crow Pose is the threshold to an arm balance practice. To begin, squat down with your hands on the floor and place your knees on the back or the side of your upper arms. Squeeze into the arms for support and inner thigh strength. Lift up one foot at a time until you can balance on your arms. Place a pile of blankets under your head just in case the first few hundred attempts don't go well.

Grace	Pose	Grit
On floor, lift the head and shoulders	Boat Pose	Arms extended, legs straight and off the floor
Downward Dog	Handstand at wall	In the middle of the room
Head resting on a block	Crow Pose	Straighten the arms

Fearlessness is not being unafraid. Fearlessness is being very afraid and doing it anyway.

To see a video of these poses, go to
www.YogaDownload.com

Fearless After Fifty: Practical Advice
Finding Our Faith

Easy and inexpensive

- Get into nature. Nothing says, "Miracle" like our natural world.

- Try something that scares you: a new food, a frightening movie, a challenging yoga pose.

- Tell someone your dreams and desires.

- Find books by some of our favorite spiritual authors: Anne Lamott, Pema Chödrön, Ram Dass, Deepak Chopra, Jack Canfield and more. The list is endless.

More ... money, time and focus

- Visit one of the natural wonders in your area.

- Charter a boat or take a rafting trip. Find the rivers, lakes, streams or oceans of our world.

- Take an intermediate yoga workshop. You can totally do it!

- Try Stand Up Yoga, or SUP, on a paddleboard. It's wobbly and fun.

- Wear a smallish bathing suit in public. This can be empowering.

All in!
- Sign up for an inversion yoga retreat or workshop.
- Find a retreat center in a place that's more challenging like Machu Picchu, the Amazon Rainforest, or the White Cliffs of Dover.
- Plan a trip to see one of the Seven Natural Wonders of the World, like the Grand Canyon, or travel to the Rocky Mountains, Alaska, Mt. Kilimanjaro or any place that makes you marvel.
- Climb a mountain or take scuba diving or snorkeling lessons.
- Sign up for a mountain bike trip, or hike or bike a foreign country.
- Do the thing that scares you the most. Tackle a phobia. Call an estranged friend.

Five
Be the Change

To be fully alive, fully human, and completely awake
is to be continually thrown out of the nest.
~ Pema Chödrön

Aging is like a great adventure. Just when we think we have
something figured out, everything changes and we have no
choice but to change along with it. To be fearless is to be okay
with the things we cannot control. With practice we might
even learn to embrace any kind of uncertainty in life. George
Bernard Shaw reminds us, "Progress is impossible without
change, and those who cannot change their minds cannot
change anything."

Take our friend Missy, 51, who was undergoing dramatic
shifts in 2016. She had her first grandchild, she was back in
the workforce, and her health and body were not the same.
She was gaining weight and feeling sluggish. Her yoga practice
was, in her words, "in the dumps."

"My instinct was to do more of what I've always done," she
confessed. Since yoga was her daily movement, she began
practicing up to twice a day. But instead of giving her increased
vitality, she felt drained. After a few months, she decided to try
something different. "You will be so proud of me," she told
Michelle one day. "I'm going to get out of my zip code," which
is one way of saying, try something new.

"I'm going to enter a body competition," Missy said. "I have a trainer. I have workout videos. I'm going to exercise, eat right, and in three months I'm going to get on a stage in a bikini." Whoa. She was right. Not many of us would choose midlife to get on a stage in a bikini. But she was definitely going to be the change she desired.

The Zip Code

Our zip code is like one big nest. It is more than where we live. It is the space where we feel comfortable. We can feather and fluff it. But eventually we have to leave it.

"Contentment can be the conundrum of change," Desiree admits, "while discontent can motivate us to do something we might not ordinarily do."

How to Know If You're Either Cozy or Caught in Your Zip Code

You are *Cozy* if ...

- Everything is working out great.
- You are content and happy.
- You want for nothing.
- You would rate your health as terrific.
- You have a gazillion friends and a few very good ones.
- You get along with your entire family.
- You are spiritually supported.
- You are materially comfortable enough.
- You wake up every day excited and happy to be you.

You are *Caught* if ...

- Things are not so great.
- You feel alone or lonely.
- Your health is meh.
- Your exercise routine is repetitive and your body is on autopilot.
- You eat the same foods every day.
- You've practiced the same yoga with the same teachers for twenty years.
- You often say, "I can't," or "I shouldn't," or "I used to."
- You are reluctant to try new things.
- Your excuses sound lame, even to you.
- The last time you "played," you were in grade school.
- You've accepted changes you don't like, because "it's the way it is."
- The last time you felt thrilled or terrified was in a previous decade.

We may think we've feathered our nest until it's just perfect. We like our routines! We are creatures of habit and seek out comfort. But what we fail to realize is that while we're snuggling in, we are changing nonetheless. Our body, mind and spirit are continuing to age and now have different needs. One day we wake up and the scale may indicate something shocking. One day we bend over and our back suddenly spasms.

These things didn't happen overnight. They occurred over a period of years while we were unconsciously going through the motions of our life. Change is constantly happening, even if we're not paying attention.

Just like it's hard to get out of a warm bed on a brisk morning, it's hard to leave our comfy nest. Humans are famously adverse to discomfort, so much so that we invented 700-thread count sheets. To move on, we have to be highly motivated. We have to want the new thing much more than what holds us back. We have to want it so much that we are willing to get uncomfortable, to get silly, to feel sore, and to do absolutely anything to find it. We have to be willing to face our fears.

Missy wanted a change so badly that she was willing to stand on a stage in a bikini to find it. That's fearlessness.

"Everything we want," Desiree tells us, "is just on the other side of what we're willing to do. It's not enough to embrace change. We have to be willing to make it happen."

Demo Day

Every home renovation begins with demo day. In yoga, transformation begins with destruction. You must dismantle something old before you can build something new. You don't want to build on old patterns. You want a clean slate. That's hard, especially if we are not conscious of the habit we've created.

Hinduism has a deity dedicated to destruction, Shiva. If you want to create change and transformation, then you would ask Shiva for help. His job is to obliterate, clear out, and erase anything that does not serve. He is basically a whirling dervish, a one-man demolition derby. He once took out an entire forest simply by dancing.

The habit we need to uproot and eradicate is the habit of "no." Many of us have built a lifetime on saying "no." We may have come to it later in life when we felt a little weaker than and not as capable as we once were. It is so much easier to believe we can't than to fathom that we can. It is easier to stay in our zip code than explore new territory. It is safer to be stuck until we can't stand it anymore. So how do we overcome a lifetime of "no"? It begins with consciousness. You must see it, know it, and deal with it to conquer it.

Notice the Habit of No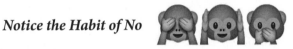

Carry a small journal or notebook.

- *Every time you say "no," write it down.*
- *Every time you think "no," write it down.*
- *Every time you hear "no," write it down.*
- *Every time you think you cannot do something, write it down.*
- *Every time you see something you cannot have, write it down.*
- *Every time a friend is doing something that you want to do, write it down.*
- *Every time something negative comes out of your mouth, write it down.*

After a week you should start to see a pattern. Please note that we're not trying to undo the habit just yet. We're just trying to see it. A habit is virtually invisible and involuntary. Certain habits are good, such as brushing our teeth, or looking both ways before we cross a street. But this habit of saying or thinking "no" holds us back. Consciousness is the way forward.

By the time we reach midlife our habits can become deeply ingrained. We've had years or decades to create a worldview. Are we funny? Are we serious? Are we who we are supposed to be? But most importantly, are we stuck?

When we find ourselves saying no to opportunities that ignite a teeny tiny spark within us, and we're not even sure why, then we are trapped in a cycle that eventually makes us smaller. We are turning away from life's exciting chances for a giggle, a smile, a new understanding, a new friend, and even a potentially negative experience. We're afraid of not winning, yet if we're not winning, we're probably learning.

It all starts with changing the habit of "no." Start with a funeral.

Burn Baby, Burn

There's nothing quite like a fire ceremony to burn out unnecessary patterns.

"It's wonderful to see things that do not serve us go up in smoke," said Desiree. "It reinforces our intention to start over."

Desiree encourages participants in her retreats to let go of the thoughts that do not serve by burning these thoughts at the stake, literally. First, write on pieces of paper the thoughts that do not serve you, the doubts, the patterns that hold you back, and the things you fear. You can even write down old, hurtful relationships you no longer wish to continue. Then build a fire, the bigger the better. Lastly, toss everything in. This is similar to Shiva, starting with destruction.

"We take all the old stuff, the relationships that don't serve us, the habits and tendencies that are harmful and we let them go," she explains. "We throw the papers on the fire and watch everything go up in smoke."

There is nothing like a ritual fire to say goodbye to old habits. You don't try to ignore them, because they will probably come back. You want them to burn, to cease and desist. Then you can start anew. Anyone can do this at home. You do not need a campfire or a group of people to support you. Simply write down what you are choosing to put an end to, and burn it in a fireplace or an old metal can. It is extremely cathartic.

Start Over with Yes

Once your demo day is complete, you are ready to build a new habit. At first, a new pattern will feel awkward. But just because something feels uncomfortable doesn't mean it's wrong. It just means you are trying on new things, having new experiences. Not all new things will feel right for you, right away, and this is okay. Trying on different patterns and habits serves two purposes: first, you will train yourself to consider "yes." Second, you may discover something you like. Think of it as kissing frogs. Any little frog could be a prince, but most will probably just be frogs. We are trying to learn the new habit of saying "yes" and embracing the awkward in life.

You will never know if you like something unless you try it. You will not know if a new activity or food is wonderful unless you take a nibble. You could miss out on a new friend unless you say "okay" for lunch. But most of all, you will change, whether you like it or not. Aging is changing; you have a chance to make it better if you stay open to new experiences and say "yes."

Where on earth do we start after half of a century doing things the old way? We always start where we are. Accept invitations. Try a different restaurant. Go to a museum, or a concert. Take a drive to another town. Attend a lecture. Try Zumba with a friend, or aerial yoga, or kickboxing. Why not?

Learning to try new things, and get out of our box is not just potentially fun. It's mandatory to keep us young, mentally sharp, and physically fit. Celebrate every single yes.

How to Practice Yes

In a journal, record every yes. Write down:

- *If you had lunch with a new friend.*
- *If you volunteered somewhere new.*
- *If you tried an unfamiliar activity, food, or yoga posture.*
- *If you had a new experience.*
- *If you said "yes."*
- *If you said, "maybe," give yourself half a point.*
- *If you assumed something was good, instead of bad.*
- *If you laughed when you could have cried.*

Yoga Is a Change Agent

If saying "no" is an unconscious pattern, then yoga is the change agent. The philosophy and the practice of yoga are meant to wake us up, and designed to guide us through transformation.

When we practice, we learn to pay attention. We are noticing and sometimes controlling the breath, which before yoga was an unconscious reflex. We are careful with every muscle and body part. We intentionally place ourselves into poses. We are waking up our bodies, minds and spirits. We see our habits more clearly so we can change them.

Simply being on the mat is enough to bring clarity to our lives. There is no chance of falling into a pattern of doing things by rote. And if you become bored, well then, there's always more. It could take a lifetime to learn the intricacies of the easy poses and to master all the harder poses.

Dharma Mittra, a teacher in New York, photographed himself in 1,350 poses when he was in midlife. There is even a new book called, *2100 Asanas*. There are enough yoga poses that you should never get bored. There is enough subtlety in the easiest poses that you can continue to learn something new each time. With guidance and gumption, you have the opportunity to say, "yes" every single time you are on the mat!

Michelle learned to say "yes" in yoga. She was used to being the tightest one in the room; it took her almost a decade to touch her toes. "When it happened, you could have knocked me over with a feather," she said. "What a delightful surprise."

Then one day her teacher asked her to demonstrate a backbend. "I'm not backbend girl," she replied to him, because her back was still stiff as a board.

"What kind of yogi is that?" he answered.

All of a sudden Michelle saw that her habit of no was still deeply rooted in her psyche. After all, what was the worst thing that could happen? Her pose wouldn't be pretty? She would get stuck? The teacher would have to call 911? If she refused to try, then she was already stuck, and that's not how she wanted to live her life. So she did the pose.

If you want to be more adventurous in life, if you want to change an unconscious habit, then yoga can be the practice for choosing "yes."

"I'm not on my mat for the exercise," Michelle said. "I'm here for the transformation. We don't get on our mats because we want to be better at yoga. We get on our mats so we can be better at life."

What holds us back? Mostly it is fear. We may be afraid of looking ridiculous or stupid. We may be afraid we won't succeed. We might be afraid that we will get hurt. Caution is important, but when it holds us back from perfectly attainable goals, then it's fear and it comes from our minds. Ego, which lives in the mind, has the job to keep us safe. After all, if the body is damaged or destroyed, then the mind would lose its comfy home. So ego works 24-7 to keep itself safe in its zip code.

The mind is not usually our friend. It is our "meddle-in-law."

The Psychology of Fear

One of the largest components of learning to deal with change is learning to deal with fear and the unknown. Human beings are hardwired for fear. Our minds are afraid of what can harm us, what we do not understand, and what can separate us from the herd. Fear is not just the thing we fear itself, but actually the thing we need to pay attention to.

Feeling anxious, apprehensive, and scared are part of the human experience. Most fears exist as a basic survival mechanism like a fear of heights since we cannot fly! If we fall from a great height we will get hurt or die. Fear of water exists because we can drown. Fear of a large animal stems from our ancestors' experience of being eaten by large animals. Fear is part of who we are.

According to Dr. Karl Albrecht,[14] our fears boil down to five basic categories:

- *Extinction* – The fear of annihilation or ceasing to exist. It is more than just the "fear of death." It is a "primary existential anxiety" in all normal humans.

- *Mutilation* – The fear of losing a part of our body; of having our boundaries invaded, or of losing the integrity and use of any organ, body part, or natural function.

- *Loss of Autonomy* – The fear of being immobilized, paralyzed, restricted, enveloped, overwhelmed, entrapped, imprisoned, smothered, or controlled by circumstances. It is sometimes known as claustrophobia, but it also extends to social interactions and relationships.

- *Separation* – The fear of abandonment, rejection, and loss of connectedness—of becoming a non-person, not wanted, respected, or valued by anyone else. This is why the "silent treatment" can have a devastating psychological effect on the targeted person.

- *Ego-death* – The fear of humiliation, shame, or any other mechanism of profound self-disapproval that threatens the loss of integrity of the Self. This fear

---

[14] Karl Albrecht, PhD, *Psychology Today*, March 22, 2012.

is of the shattering of one's constructed sense of lovability, capability, and worthiness.

We Are Human, Now What?

Even though fear is a part of the human condition, the question becomes how do we live with it? How do we not let it hold us back from our best lives? How do we become beings of "yes," not held back by our fears? Certain fears are part of our survival mechanism, and some are entrenched by our habits.

If some of our concerns are hardwired, and some are a habit, does it matter which is which? If the point of being afraid is to wake us up, then does it truly matter? Because whether or not we are terrified because of a biological reason, or a childhood phobia, or just an established habit, all of it serves to wake us up. What matters is how we learn to work with it, honor it, and not let it hold us back.

As Desiree says, "Love is stronger than fear."

Inversions Make Us Fearless

To be fearless, we have to practice courage. We want to take baby steps into bravery, not giant leaps. A giant leap is admittedly terrifying and possibly unwise. Creeping up to the edge and peeking over is a safer approach to overcoming our fears.

Many poses help us practice fearlessness, but none more so than inversions. We should have a healthy fear of going upside down because it is an innate fear of getting hurt. It is also a reflexive response to doing something new. After all, most of us spend our lives on our feet and not our hands.

Therefore, if we practice it, theoretically, we can move past it.

The practice of yoga is the practice of moving into consciousness, while becoming comfortable with discomfort. Essentially, we are animals, yet the practice of being human is like the practice of yoga: we want to move beyond our "animal nature." We want to rise above the animal "fight or flight" reflex. Rather than react unconsciously, we seek to reason and act responsibly. We have the power to think beyond our biology. When we meet a new person, we don't (or shouldn't!) snarl and bite. We use our senses to determine if we are in danger or not.

Life is a constant exercise between the "yes" and the "no," the play between being afraid and being brave, and the space between habit and practice. Living fearlessly is the choice between living either an unconscious or conscious life. We don't want to miss any of it. We are willing to take the good with the bad, so we can enjoy it all.

Yoga heightens our ability to use our rational nature and practice the "yes" in life. Every time we try something we don't think we can do on the mat, it is a teeny, tiny affirmation that we can do the same in life. We may be animals, but as human animals we can be fully awake and aware, and we can rise above our fear. To be fearless is to say, "yes" above the unconscious habit of "no." To be fearless after fifty is not to be unafraid. It is to practice something that scares us, it is to be conscious and awake, it is to be willing to take the good with the bad, so we don't miss a moment of our lives.

The physical sequence, breath, and philosophy of yoga work together to wake us up. We learn to pause, to think, to consider, and to act in a higher, more reasonable and resolved manner. We learn to destroy with vigor the things that do not serve us. We embrace transformation and use our yoga practice to train ourselves to think first, react second.

In this way, yoga helps us *be* the change.

The normal human experience is to react without thinking, it is the fight or flight reflex. Thinking before reacting is not easy. It's not even natural, which is why people say to count to 10 or take a deep breath. The normal human experience is to react, overreact, take offense, argue, rebut, and seek to control the things we cannot control. Yet we want to live a life that's not the normal human experience. We want to find a peaceful mind, happiness in our spirit, and rise above our fears, especially as we age.

"I don't want the 'normal' human experience."
~ **Desiree Rumbaugh**

It's not your imagination that if you feel more afraid these days, it's probably because you are older. According to the Geriatric Mental Health Foundation, aging increases anxieties, fears and worries. In fact, the kind of paralyzing anxiety that includes phobias, terrors, and obsessions afflict older people more than the average young person. If you had these tendencies when you were young and strong, they do not get better. Unless treated, they get worse.

Terrors That Increase with Age

- *Obsessions*
- *Depression*
- *Panic Disorders*
- *Social Phobias*
- *Agoraphobia*
- *Post-Traumatic Stress Disorder (PTSD)*
- *Generalized Anxiety Disorder*

What causes us to become so afraid? Theories abound and they include increasing isolation, illness, and untreated PTSD from events that happened earlier in our lives. However, it doesn't have to be this way. Just being aware that this is part of the aging experience will help us throw these fears into the fire, so to speak.

A Life Without Worry Takes Work

Regrets make us sad, yet they are also another way we avoid transformation. Why deal with the present when we can spend our days in the past? If the present time is awkward and uncomfortable, if it means taking responsibility for our lives and our actions, well then why not spend time in the past where we know how things turned out? Regrets can be a kind of escapism. Regrets, like fears, also increase with age.

Apparently, if we don't come to terms with the happenstance of our life, those little doubts and misgivings don't actually disappear. They grow like mold until the tentacles of remorse reach out and suffocate us.

Holidays

For those of us who have suffered a tremendous loss, or who have experienced trauma and regret, holidays can be the worst. They bring up all our shortcomings. They highlight the fact that our family relationships are often problematic. The pressure is on to be merry, but the truth is that holidays can be lonely. Rather than looking around the table and seeing who is there, we stare into the past to see who is missing.

"After I lost Brandon, I learned to live with the pain," said Desiree. "Yet at holidays and family gatherings, I am always aware of his absence. The first few years were the most difficult for me. I couldn't bear the celebration of any holidays or events. I dropped out of life and was mired in sadness. But after three full years of this suffering, I realized my pain had become a habit. I then had to choose to look at those experiences in a different way. I realized life would be pretty terrible if every single person who suffered a loss, or who had a difficult relationship with their family, opted to no longer celebrate life. So I made a conscious decision that to celebrate was to live for others, if not yet for myself."

"From time to time we may indulge in magical thinking wondering how things might have been," Desiree continues. "But as I become aware that it is my mind causing my pain, I learn I can change the channel. I tell my heart that it's okay to miss him. It's okay to feel the pain, yet it would be a shame to spend so much time stuck in that sadness that I miss the perfectly wonderful moments at hand."

Desiree is not alone. Who doesn't have regret? A study conducted by the National Institutes of Health (May 2008) revealed that the biggest regrets in life are:

Career *Leisure*
Self-development
Education
PARENTING
Romance

It is good to know our misery has company!

Studies show that the worst regrets are directly linked to our perceived opportunity. So, if we felt we had no chance, none whatsoever, then we probably have fewer regrets around that subject. For example, if we lost a job opportunity to someone with much more experience, *whatever*. But the times when we could have made a better decision, or been a better parent, or been more compassionate in a relationship, these things can haunt us.

Parenting can be the worst regret. Who wouldn't be a better parent after having done it once or twice? But part of the experience, we are convinced, is learning to accept our limitations and forgive ourselves. We have to accept that we did the best we could, and let go of the rest. Perhaps the ultimate parenting lessons are the ones we give ourselves in forgiveness?

If the regrets that we cannot let go of, or forgive ourselves for, are directly tied to our potential opportunities, then perhaps are regrets also a way to wake us up? If you regret not finishing school, for example, is now the time? If you regret losing contact with an old friend, pick up the phone. If you regret growing apart from family, is it too late to reconnect? Can you do something that will lead to less doubt and more happiness?

Regret is nature's way of bringing our attention to something that feels unresolved. Try to be brave and face it. Rather than avoid that past experience, meditate on it. Give it time and thought and you may make peace with it, or someday throw it in the fire.

Decisions, Decisions

Decisions can also turn into regrets in disguise. If we once made a decision that we regret, it can lead us to doubt our future decisions. And where do decisions come from? The mind!

In yoga, we learn to trust our heart before we listen to the mind. If it were up to the mind, we'd never try a handstand, or look silly on our mat. So when the mind chides us, "Don't do it; you'll get hurt and leave me without a warm body," we thank it for sharing and move on.

Doubt your doubts. Decisions are just markers for moments in time. You did what you did with what you knew then. You may do it differently now, but this is now, and that was then. Don't let a decision come back to haunt you. That's part of the practice of forgiveness and moving on.

Decisions beget more decisions. They multiply and there will always be another. Don't get hung up on one, because you will miss the next one. It's like a game of tennis. If you get hung up on how you hit the last ball, you will never get the next one. Let it go and move on.

Change Is Hard, Especially for Others

When you make a huge change in your life—let's say you move, or lose a tremendous amount of weight, or suddenly found new self-confidence—the transformation doesn't just affect you. It is also a change for your immediate support group. It can be hard on us when our circle is not helpful, yet it can also reinforce our determination to stay on a new path.

Michelle is a lifetime member of Weight Watchers©, having lost a great deal of weight with the plan after she had children. It was at a meeting that her leader said, "From now on, she was going to be my one true friend," Michelle remembers. "That was because everyone else in my life was going to sabotage my efforts."

It turned out to be true! Michelle's new lifestyle and healthy eating habits were not only hard for her, but they were hard for everyone else in her life. Out of "love," friends would offer her a piece of cake, or more wine. Out of "love," they would say, "You don't have to lose weight." But it wasn't love. It was fear that the change she was embracing was going to somehow adversely affect them! So once you decide on making a change, you may have to help others around you to accept it as well.

If we try on something new, we can't expect the same enthusiasm from friends. Your transformation may not be theirs. Your friends may say that doing yoga is crazy. Or your family may feel that recognizing Buddhist philosophies of Karma is against their religion. If you begin eating a plant-based diet, expect some push back from the hamburger helpers. If you resolve to live a more "lightened" life, then expect others to offer you wine and cake. You will have to make a choice. Do you help others who are resisting change to make a change with you? Or do you leave them be? Can you accept their path? Do you simply follow a new path on your own? Do you model new habit patterns for other people? Can those with an alternative path still be friends with you?

A question that sometimes drives me hazy:
Am I, or are the others crazy?"
~ **Albert Einstein**

When the Change Is Not So Pretty

Youth certainly seems to have it all: energy, enthusiasm, health, and a boundless appetite for adventure. It is natural that our egos attach our sense of pride and self-esteem to the traits we possessed as younger people. So then how do we accept the things we don't want to accept, such as slowing down, illness, injury, or just what we see when we look in the mirror?

Perhaps we were once proud of our physical strength, beauty, shape and/or size. We may have been geniuses, and now we can't remember where we put the car keys. Our brains spend more time searching for the names of old things than coming up with new ideas. We may have been naturally thin and now we carry more around the middle. We may have been strong and now we struggle with opening a can. We may have been flexible and now we can't touch our toes. Some of us can't even see them!

How do we learn to thrive when so many things are different? We want to embrace change. We don't deny it. Yet that doesn't mean we have to always like it.

The Nature of Suffering

The center of Buddhist thought is the concept of suffering. Suffering is inevitable, so we want to understand it, make peace with it, and live with it.

The ego is the part of our being that doesn't like change and attaches to suffering. However, we can't very well throw it into the fire with the other habits that do not serve us, can we? Ego is part of who we are, and it has an important job of keeping us safe; when it is held in balance, the ego provides self-esteem. And yet ego attaches to the silliest of things, like how we look in jeans or a new wrinkle on our face. Finding happiness has to be about finding a way to live with what we cannot change.

Aging brings about certain changes. Our bones become more brittle. It takes work to keep our muscles strong. Weight starts to pool in the most unfortunate of places. So what are we going to do? Do we want to spend 95% of our time crying about what we cannot change? Suffering in this way is entirely our choice. Yet suffering exists because we attach to our desires.

Suffering is part of life. We want to live in Disneyland, but unfortunately it's not a real place. Life is change and is temporary, and still we attach to things hoping they are permanent. Guess what? We cause most of our own suffering! In an unconscious way we've chosen to attach our happiness to things we have no control over. What is wrong with us?

If we allow our egos to attach to the things that will change, such as the beauty of our physical form, then we will be miserable. However, if you can find something about you that you like, such as your sense of humor, or your intelligence, or how you can make pie, then you will be joyous. If you appreciate the light in your own eyes and how happiness over the years has given you a smile line, then you are making peace with change.

We can end suffering by practicing non-attachment. Can we really do this? Can we live in the present moment without spending time on regrets from the past? Can we stop wishing for things in the future? Living in the present and being content is perhaps the hardest transformation of all. Happiness, in many ways, is the belief that things are the way they are supposed to be.

Our ability to cope with change, including the changes we may not appreciate, indicates our willingness to grow. If we want to evolve, to learn and to transform, then each experience, good and bad, moves us along the path. "To live fully is to be always in no-man's-land," teaches Pema Chödrön, "experiencing each moment as completely new and fresh."

To be continually thrown out of our zip code, or our nest, is to be fully alive.

Add More Play To Your Day

So far all this change sounds like a lot of work. We have to wake up, be uncomfortable, throw things in a fire, and start new habits. We have to live in the present and not regret the past (good luck!). We may have to stand on a stage in a bikini, or do something else equally awkward. But there is an easier way to bring about cognitive change in our lives.

Science has proven beyond any doubt that play is beneficial to the developing brain. In 1964, neuroscientists led by Marion Diamond discovered that rats that were allowed play learned quicker and went further in a maze than rats that didn't. Further, researchers discovered that rats with "enrichment" play had thicker cerebral cortices than "impoverished" rats. If given a choice, what kind of rat do you want to be? One with a bigger, enriched brain, or a depleted one? Being impoverished or lacking doesn't sound so good to us.

Exercise alone has been shown to boost our feel good hormones (endorphins), and lower our stress hormones (cortisol and adrenaline). But there are specific neurons that fire with free play. Any structured exercise routine, such as PE class, will not reap the same benefits as recess.

Play sparks creativity, and creativity is the key to brain development.

"As adults, we can still access that kid inside us and infuse our days with joyful, creative energy," explains Desiree. "One of the joys of yoga is to keep a fresh perspective, to be willing to try new things, and maintain a beginner's mind. Yet because it's such a simple idea, the importance and depth of it frequently gets underestimated and overlooked."

"We want to turn fear into fun," she says.

Some of us may need help to exercise the "fun" muscle. Life can get serious and get us down. Here are some tips on how to get started having fun again.

A Play Primer for the Fun-Challenged

- **Be willing to laugh when you "fail."**
  You are not supposed to be "good" at playing.
  If you take yourself seriously when you are trying
  to have fun, you are missing the point. Tell your
  ego to calm down during recess.

- **Failure is relative.**
  What many see as failure is actually only feedback.
  Try to see the joyful experience of falling down,
  getting up and starting over. It takes the sting out
  of life.

- **Believe you can do it.**
  It's amazing what we can do when we think we can
  do it. Speak to yourself kindly. Kids believe in
  superheroes. Engage your own superhero with
  your attitude.

- **Be willing to look silly.**
  Our culture ties pride to appearance. When children
  play, the last thing on their mind is how they look.
  Make joy more important than your image, and
  you'll inspire others to find joy, too.

- **Be your unique, amazing self.**
  Play is a time to let the editor go. Don't second guess.
  Don't rehearse or prepare. Don't over analyze the
  rules. That is such a grown up thing to do. Approach
  a task with exuberance and see what happens.

- **Shake it up.**
  Play is a chance to do things differently. Walk
  backwards. Brush your teeth with the "other" hand.
  Speak Pig Latin. Eat dessert first. Whatever it is,
  embrace the dissimilar.

- **Observe younger generations.**
  Interacting with children is revitalizing since they
  have a way of seeing things differently. Try on their
  perspective in order to renew your own.

- **Toys R for us, too.**
  Remember that hula-hoop? Why not try it again?
  How about snowshoes? Snowshoeing gets you
  outdoors in winter. Learn a new, playful skill and
  watch your brain get fat and happy.

Dharma Not Drama

One of the best lessons from accessing play is that it teaches
us how to separate our actions from the result of those actions.
We want to play because it is fun. We want to try new things
and look silly to take a break from being an adult all the time.
We want a big brain, a happy spirit, and a healthy body. We
want to laugh. It shouldn't matter as much if we win at the
game; it's truly just that we play it. Someone probably told us
that when we were growing up.

"Play is something done for its own sake," said Dr. Stuart
Brown, director of the National Institute for Play.[15] "Play
is voluntary, it's pleasurable, it offers a sense of engagement,
it takes you out of time. And the act itself is more important
than the outcome."

In yoga, this lesson is taught within the *Bhagavad Gita*, an
epic poem inside the *Mahabharata*, dating as early as the fifth
century BCE. The *Bhagavad Gita* tells the story of Arjuna the
warrior, who is trying to understand his destiny. Arjuna learns
that someone performs his duty, simply for duty's sake. If you
do something only to reap a reward, you are missing the point
and will likely be disappointed. If you do it just to do it, you

---

[15] Story by Sami Yenigun, National Public Radio: All Things Considered, August 6,
2014.

will always "win" at life. "You have a right to your actions, but never to the fruit of your actions," the Gita teaches us.

If you do the duties of a parent only to create a perfect child, then you will likely be disappointed. Parent for parenting's sake, and for the love of your child. If you exercise only to get a super model's figure, you will be disappointed. Exercise for exercise's sake to take care of your body. If you play only to win, you will surely be disappointed. Play for play's sake, and you will be rewarded by feeling enlivened in mind and spirit.

Creativity, Culture and Curiosity - The Three Cs.

Another path to lead us around the things we fear and into the path of transformation is to cultivate our creativity. We have two brains, the right and the left. Both need nurturing to continue to grow.

In Elizabeth Gilbert's book, *Big Magic: Creative Living Beyond Fear*, she contends that what holds us back from living our best life is fear, and the way to get around this monkey in the middle is by being creative.

"Do whatever brings you to life," she writes. "Follow your own fascinations, obsessions, and compulsions. Trust them. Create whatever causes a revolution in your heart."

We are after a revolution in our lives. We encourage you to embrace change by any means, whether it is through conscious play, creativity or participating in a cultural event. Whatever we can do to stimulate our curiosity will keep us alive and awake. Creativity, culture and curiosity all work to develop the right side of the brain. These things will keep our perspectives fresh and current.

"But ladies, I'm not the creative type!"

Yes, we've heard that, but actually, it's not true. Every human being has a creative side, and we have to work to keep it alive. If you've never been creative, then developing this skill doesn't have to be overwhelming. You only need to pay attention to what gets your attention. Creativity can stem from a tiny, curious inkling. Explore it. Enjoy it. Know that it is stimulating curiosity in a non-fearful way. We want to explore change and take baby steps into bravery without awakening the fear-monkey in the room. It's just the tiniest of adventures to keep us in the game.

How to Foster Creativity

- **Write**
  Start every day with old-fashioned handwriting.
  Make a list, write in a journal or simply jot down
  what you see out the window. Handwriting stimulates
  the creative part of our brain, and studies show that
  we are forgetting how to do it by using computers
  too much!

- **Support the Arts**
  Make a culture date once a month with a friend or
  by yourself. Choose a museum, art gallery, play,
  or musical performance to attend. Support a show
  at your local high school or community college.
  Seek out Community Theater. You get the idea.

- **Paint**
  You do not have to be Renoir to paint something.
  There are a slew of coloring books on the market
  lately because drawing, coloring and painting have

been shown to stimulate the brain. Refinish a piece of furniture. Paint a wall. Make a picture. Decorate a vase with flowers. Find something and change it.

- **Find a Hobby**
  Any hobby will suffice. Make something. Try gardening, pottery, papier-mâché, embroidery, model airplanes, woodcarving, or knitting. There are classes at senior centers, rec centers and schools. Make something new by hand, and you will discover a change in your spirit.

Some Things You Can't Change

Now that you are excited to get out there and make some change happen, we want to counsel you there are certain things best left alone. There are three things that are a complete waste of time for you to try and change. We know this for sure:

Three Things You CANNOT Change:

- *Life. It is not fair.*
- *People. They will let you down.*
- *Having control. Sometimes life turns out differently, but it could be better.*

Life is not fair. Sorry, but it's true. Don't try to change that. You can't.

People will disappoint you. They are not saints. They are humans. They are imperfect. It's up to you to forgive and move on. It's not up to them to change. If you don't like the way things are, you are the only one who can change it.

Lastly, we don't have that much control over the way things turn out. Life will take a few strange twists and turns we never saw coming. There are no guarantees. But honestly, it could be much better. You have to live all the way to the end of the story to know for sure how it will end.

Three Things you CAN Change:

- *Change your mind or attitude.*
- *Change your spirit.*
- *Change your health: physical, mental and spiritual.*

Change your attitude and get your mind under control. We cannot say it enough. Life is entirely how you look at it. Living a problem-free life is entirely within your power, and it starts between the ears. Change what you can, try to play more, be creative and curious, and learn to live with the rest.

Change your spirit by feeding it. Have faith. Invite abundance. Make friends. If you are unhappy, maybe it's time for therapy? Perhaps our phobias and fears are a means to wake us up to deal with the underpinnings of our psychosis? It's never too late to be happy. It's a choice, often requiring courage, and a path we can follow.

Change your health. Make your health a priority. You can't be of service to anyone else if you are needy, frail, and unwell. Make sure you are doing everything possible to live a pain free life. We are on a never-ending journey of living well. If one therapy isn't working, try another. Get out of your zip code and try anything, something, to find your best self.

A Word About That Change ... The Big Change

Menopause naturally occurs at midlife to both men and women. While female menopause is the eventual end of one's menstrual cycle, male menopause is associated with a drop in hormones including testosterone. Both male and female menopauses are a big, *huge*, change. While some of us sail right through this time in our lives, *others do not*.

One of us, Desiree, kept right on going through that time. She kept up her stamina, adjusted her diet to add more protein and nutrition, and generally felt fine. Michelle—not so much. Starting in her 40s, she was sick for nearly seven years. She could not sleep, had difficulty thinking, gained weight, lost her balance, suffered anxiety, depression, and debilitating panic attacks. She had numerous medical interventions, but not one doctor identified the source—menopause.

Menopause may be a natural state, yet there is no such thing as a normal passage through this time. It is a very unique experience. So if you feel that you are not "just sailing through it," we urge you to seek expert help. Use this time to become more aware of your body and your personal needs. Put yourself first. Seek out treatment, new exercise routines, new yoga classes, and new perspectives outside traditional medicine.

Michelle finally got help. It involved hormones, a change in her sleep patterns, and a blend of Eastern and Western medicine. Do not, we repeat, do not give up until you get the answers that bring relief.

Time Is the Best Change Agent

Steve Jobs once said that death is the greatest change agent. It brings term limits to what we can accomplish in life. So getting older should motivate us to finish what we started. Aging, with all of its complexities, bizarre adjustments, strengthening and weakening of various systems, has the power to bring about our greatest transformations.

Aging can make us better human beings. We might seek out the answers to long held questions about our behaviors, our fears, and our willingness to change our focus to what matters, and practice non-attachment to the things that don't matter.

"Fear is a natural reaction to moving closer to the truth," explains Pema Chödrön. We can take baby steps to bravery. We can use our fears to wake up, to move closer to the certainty of who we are, and to be the change before it changes us.

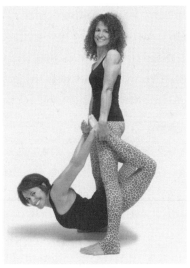

Yogis Playing in a Swing

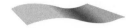

The Practice:
Shouldering On!

We carry the weight of the world and all the change it brings on our shoulders. By midlife, our shoulders need love as well. They can become tight and rounded, putting our shoulder girdle at risk for injury. Regaining our mobility relieves pain and stress and protects that shoulder girdle for life.

Stretching
- **Standing Wall Stretch**
  Face a wall and place your hand firmly on it in front of you. Keeping the arm and wrist straight, slowly turn away from the wall into the center of the room.
  Now stand with your side to a wall, reach back behind you with one arm and press your hand into the wall. Slowly turn your body away from the wall to stretch the inner shoulder and pectoral muscles.

- **Belt Stretch**
  Holding the ends of a yoga strap or belt, raise the arms overhead. Gently stretch from side to side, front to back.

Strengthening
- **Rear Deltoid Builder, Reverse Plank, *Purvottanasana***
  Sit on a mat with your legs bent and feet on the floor. Place your hands directly behind you, fingers forward,

shoulder distance apart. Lift your ribcage and shoulders, then bend your elbows and squeeze the bottom tips of your shoulder blades toward each other to lift your heart. Avoid throwing your head back. This pose can also be done with straight legs..

Yoga Poses for Shoulders

- **Yoga Push Up,** *Chaturanga*
  This pose can be a shoulder strengthener, but if done incorrectly, it can cause damage. We recommend you seek out personal instruction. From a plank position with arms straight, slowly bend the arms until they are at 90 degrees. The shoulder blades should be on the back. The core keeps you connected and steady. The elbows might be near the body or slightly outward in order to place the shoulders on the back. If you have pain, stop immediately.

- **Cobra,** *Bhujangasana*
  Cobra is a stretch and a strengthener. Lying on your belly, press all ten toenails down and engage your legs including your glutes. Place your hands beside your rib cage and rest your forehead on the floor. Lift the heads of your arm bones up toward your ears and then away from the floor. Squeeze the bottom tips of your shoulder blades toward each other. Tighten the muscles of your corset and curl up into a backbend. Avoid throwing your head back. Keep your elbows bent to

increase the articulation of your vertebrae especially in the upper back.

Grace	Pose	Grit
Knees on ground	*Chaturanga*	Hold in plank for 5 breaths
On Belly, squeeze shoulders	Cobra	Thighs off the ground in Upward Facing Dog
Sitting upright	*Purvottanasana*	Straight legs, hold 5 breaths

For a change, try laughing your way to enlightenment.
To see a video of these poses, go to
www.YogaDownload.com

Fearless After Fifty: Practical Advice
Finding Our Inner Child

Easy and inexpensive

- Babysit or borrow a child for a day! Go to the park, swing and slide and enjoy.

- Play in nature. Do yoga in a park.

- Volunteer at a community center or preschool. Children's delight is highly contagious.

- Get sidewalk chalk and make a hopscotch board!

More ... money, time and focus

- Go to a creative store and make pottery, art, paint on canvas, etc.

- Instead of buying something you need, make it.

- Take a sewing, pottery, or art class.

- Rediscover Play-Doh™.

- Begin a knitting, needlepoint, or other creative project.

All in!

- Add play to your bucket list. Try skydiving or hot air ballooning.

- Set aside time each day for coloring. There are a plethora of adult coloring books available.

- Set up a table for Legos™ or do a puzzle.

- Make an adult "play date." Seriously, do it.

Six
Warrior Heal Thyself

No amount of self-improvement
can make up for any lack of self-acceptance.
~ Robert Holden, PhD

Pain is like a doorbell. When it rings, we need to answer it.

Some of us may think that having pain is a normal part of life and part of the human condition. And it's true that injury happens, but it doesn't need to last longer than necessary. Discomfort of all types could be present to get our attention so we can make the necessary changes to heal ourselves once and for all. "Discomfort is the teacher," said the philosopher Lee Lozowick.

According to the American Pain Foundation, nearly 50 million Americans live with chronic, pervasive, inescapable pain. But wait, it can get worse and it usually does. Up to 60% of us do not seek medical or other kinds of help to get rid of it, according to the American Osteopathic Association.

Why is this? Why would we not pay attention when our bell is being rung? Aging, with all of its changes in the body, often feels like one big wake-up call. Could it be that we think experiencing pain is part of the normal human experience?

We've said it before, and we'll say it again: *We don't want the normal human experience!*

Illness Wakes Us Up, Too

In 2016, Desiree had to deal with an excruciating case of tinnitus, a ringing in the ears that disrupted her sleep and caused her to be temporarily unable to travel and work. "I realize that many people have to learn to live with a disability, but that doesn't mean that it is easy to do," she said.

Michelle also had a terrible, horrible, no good very bad year in which she broke five bones, fractured her neck, suffered numbness in her arms, had eye surgery, and lost her voice so that she could not teach publicly for six months. That was unpleasant, to say the least.

"From the moment we are born, we are healing," said Cat, a personal trainer in Denver. "Injury is our greatest concern as trainers because that's the one thing that has the power to make a person quit exercising."

Pain, injury, illness—anything that slows us down is not our nemesis. The real problem is ignoring it, pretending it doesn't exist. If we don't pay attention, if we give up and become immobile, then we might as well smoke a pack a day of cigarettes. Remember, sitting is the new smoking.

A Pain Poem for the Pessimistic

If we change our attitude about pain
then setbacks can be our gain.
Pain can be our teacher or guru.
It can show us what we need to do.
It can teach us what we need to know,
and it will help us heal and grow.

The life lessons in being humanly imperfect are not easy, especially to a generation that is used to succeeding and surpassing. As we age, these signs of being mortal are perhaps the most humbling messages our bodies tell us. We don't like to be "less than." We are used to kicking butt, not dragging it out of bed. Slowing down is maybe the hardest speed of all.

But when the going gets tough, the tough have to heal. Steadiness is our path through the difficult times. The measure of a yogi is taken not when we have a setback; it's taken when we rise back up and soldier on.

Listen Up

Pain is actually a path to living an awake and aware life. Therefore, we need to listen carefully to what our bodies, mind and spirit are telling us.

"In order to age fearlessly, it's crucial to study this body in which we live," Desiree points out. "Even a simple understanding of your bones, your back, how the shoulders are connected to your neck, the relationship between your hips, legs and knees, goes a long way in learning how to heal. The next time you experience pain, or are trying to fall asleep with a nagging backache, the answer might be in beginning a yoga practice. You can learn how to incrementally shift positions, or find the right alignment to ease your suffering. Breath, proper positioning, and a stress-free mind can go a long way to ease your level of pain."

Practicing yoga is living a preventative life. When we pursue yoga regularly, we become more sensitive and tuned in to our bodies. We shouldn't have to rely on a once-a-year physical checkup to know if something is going off the rails.

When we are out of sorts, or some aspect of our physical or mental fabric begins to go awry, the faster we realize it, the faster we can address it. A yogi who is attuned to their body will know immediately when something is not right and act upon it.

"Having a regular yoga practice is like having a state of the art diagnostic computer assessing your body, emotions and mind all the time," asserts Desiree. "Then you are the first to know when something is up."

Aging means we are constantly shifting, recalibrating, revising and healing. Pain and injury are tremendous consciousness-makers. When we feel great, we run around doing our regular activities and think nothing of it; it is like sleepwalking through life. But when we are in pain, we think only of that. In a way, that makes us more mindful. We are completely present, and that's a gift. Being grateful for that gift of attention is another major lesson in life.

If we are aware that we're in a constant state of "healing," and if we are determined to get back up after a setback, then there are only two mistakes we can make. One is to come back too fast or too hard. And the second is not to come back at all.

Upgrade Your Operating System

Being a yogi means being awake and aware of your body, mind and spirit. Consciousness is actually an upgrade to the standard human operating system! You will know immediately how you feel, because you are in touch with yourself. Over time you will learn to decipher if you are doing too much or too little. You will know if you have given up when you need to be getting up. The body tells us almost immediately how it feels. We just have to listen to the clues.

Desiree explains, "A regular yoga practice includes a knowledge of how the body works. So if we can do something easily one day but not the next, then we can become curious about the cause of that. Our attitude toward any body aches or twinges begins to alter. Then we can move from being passive participants in life's ups and downs to those who actively take charge of their health." Rather than merely assume, "I need to take a break," we can learn to assess. From *assume* to *assess* is a journey of consciousness, self-awareness, self-care, and empowerment.

Of course there are times when you must rest, just like there are times when you must walk, run, hop, skip, or jump. If you fracture a bone, for instance, you can't move that limb for a time. Yet you can move the rest of the body. If you have the flu you must take some time off. But you can breathe, meditate and practice steadiness in the spirit, and focused consciousness in the mind. If you have muscle soreness, do not assume you need to give that area of the body a break. You will have to assess the complexity of the pain first. A complete tear might need to rest. But most often the remedy for soreness is movement. In fact, in February of 2017, the American College of Physicians issued new guidelines for back pain stating that exercise, acupuncture, yoga, and massage might provide immediate relief.[16]

This is a sea change away from the days of old when everyone thought muscle soreness meant we had to go to bed.

"There are always ways we can work around an issue rather than letting everything go," Desiree tells us. "Injury and

---

[16] American College of Physicians, "Noninvasive Treatments for Acute, Subacute, and Chronic Low Back Pain: A Clinical Practice Guideline," 2/14/2017.

illness force us to get creative. Even when we have a broken limb there are still ways to practice yoga to safely protect that area of the body, rather than taking six weeks off from maintaining our health through daily exercise. It doesn't take long at all for us to become completely immobile—all because of one small setback."

Keeping our setbacks in perspective is the answer. The first step is always to go from assume to assess.

Make Love, Not War

Knowing when to get up rather than give up is key to staying active and vibrant. There are times when you must rest and take a break. Not listening to the messages your body sends and "pushing through" pain is as damaging as throwing in the towel. It is waging war on your body.

We are willing to bet that everyone has waged war on his or her body in one way or another, at some time in the past. If you practice yoga or exercise out of alignment, it hurts. If you overdo an activity, it hurts. If you eat poorly, or not enough, or drink too much, it hurts *and* you will pay dearly in the morning. "You cannot wage war on the body without the violence affecting the mind," said Yoga Teacher Christina Sell.

On the other hand, "If you are kind to your body, it will respond in the most incredible way," Vanda Scaravelli tells us. She practiced yoga almost daily well into her 90s. Being kind to the body is not always easy, however. It starts with being better listeners. We need to be compassionate with ourselves. As you've heard us say, pain happens for a reason: to get our attention.

When we find ourselves with illness and setbacks, it is a chance to go deeper into the practice of awareness and self-compassion. You can be wholly awake to the alignment that heals any stumbling block. You can also be filled with compassion, sympathy and steadiness; that in turn builds love for yourself. When we can manage only a tiny movement, or enjoy just the sweetest breath, it's a chance to practice letting go of expectations. We can be at peace with who we are that particular day, nothing more and nothing less.

"On the days when I'm injured or under the weather," Michelle explains, "those tend to be the days when I have the best yoga practice sessions. I never over- or under-extend myself. I seem to be the most in touch, and therefore I take better care of this body and mind and spirit. I make my healing a priority, and that is a precious gift."

The Gift That Keeps on Giving

The truth is that nothing has the potential to teach us more than a recurring or nagging injury. Many of us deal with a sore back, or an aching knee on a regular basis. Michelle has a recurring injury in her elbow sometimes called "tennis elbow."

"This set me on a journey to become more curious about my bodily alignment and how it all pieced together," she said. I am both happy and sad to say that as many times as I have had no pain, I have also re-injured my elbow. Therefore, it is a constant process of journey and discovery as we age. It keeps me very much awake and in the game, especially when I do the poses that could cause damage."

The answers, for all of us, are going to be partly in a general "correct" approach and alignment, and in what works for us as individuals. As warriors in aging, it will be up to us to heal ourselves.

Yoga as Therapy

A thousand years ago when a physical injury happened, the sages did not have Advil™ or Tylenol ™ or joint replacement surgeries. Their go-to remedy was yoga. There was no magic pill to ease their pain. They had no choice but to take excellent care of their original equipment.

Today, the pharmaceutical industry promises us a faster, better, stronger lifestyle. More than 60% of Americans take a prescription drug, according to the *Journal of the American Medical Association*. Additionally, more of us take up to six prescription drugs at a time. According to Medscape, 62% of doctor visits end with a prescription drug.

We are not saying that you shouldn't take your medicines. Not at all. Let's not be ridiculous. There are times when you must see a doctor and you absolutely must take pharmaceuticals.

What we are saying though, is that there really is no magic pill. We are going to have to do some of the hard work of healing by ourselves.

Roll Out Your Mat

In many ways yoga is an excellent therapeutic treatment for numerous bodily aches and pains. Every yoga pose has the promise to heal. As yoga teachers and practitioners, each of us has spent time pursuing the hardest poses. Desiree has both a beautiful practice and a dedicated work ethic. Michelle went after the hard poses like a trout for a fly. But here in midlife, we have both changed our attitude a bit. We no longer work for the poses. We make the poses work for us.

If you are just starting your yoga practice, or if you are working to heal your body, we want to stress the importance of finding a skilled local teacher. This is especially true when you have been injured or are in need of "repair." You want to be sure you are doing more good than harm. Everyone has to heal from time to time, and practicing with a skilled teacher, as well as an empathetic and supportive community, is often the best treatment option. In fact, you should begin by scheduling a private session to be sure you are doing the absolute best you can for your body and your individual needs.

Trauma Lives in the Body

From time to time the root of our pain isn't actually physical. Depression, trauma and stress all cause real physical symptoms that can be improved with yoga poses.

"The body keeps the score," wrote Dr. Bessel Van Der Kolk, in the book of the same title. She documents how one's physical body holds onto pain. In addition, serious neurological damage occurs from emotional trauma.

"I suffered from chronic pain in my right side, from my neck to lower back, and even down my leg. Yet no matter what kind of remedy I tried, it did not go away," Michelle explains. "When I connected this pain to a traumatic event in my childhood when my shoulder was broken, I was able to address the source, practice forgiveness, and start to heal. It might sound nutty, but it worked."

Feeling Down is Also Going Up

Depression is a source of chronic pain for many individuals. More than 19 million Americans, or almost 10% of us, suffer from depression, according to the All About Depression research group. "A heaviness of heart" was once thought to be a natural consequence of aging, but we know now that that isn't true. "Depression is a common problem among older adults, but it is *not* a normal part of aging," researchers from the NIH Senior Health division discovered.[17] "In fact, studies show that most older adults feel satisfied with their lives, despite having more illnesses or physical problems."

Mindy Greenstein and Jimmie Holland researched the phenomena of aging in their book, *Lighter As We Go* and found astonishingly that our happiest time of all is from when we are 82 to 85! Interestingly, they wrote that the saddest years are those in our midlife. We actually bottom out at 50. More of us feel down now than ever before, and the best is yet to come. But although that may be true, we have to do the work and pave the way so we can be happier at 80. It won't be handed to us; it's going to have to be hard-won.

"Being happy is not always as simple as just choosing it," Michelle points out. "It's often an act of courage." Michelle is one of those 19 million people who suffer from depression. The disorder may be called the blues, or the dumps, but it is a serious illness that affects brain chemistry. Research tells us that factors that contribute to the onset of depression include genetics, changes in hormone levels, certain medical conditions, stress, grief or difficult life circumstances, according to the Mental Health Depression Toolkit.

"I needed medication to get out of bed," Michelle said. "I tried everything: therapy, pharmaceuticals, and I was even considering more serious alternatives. I was not living the life I wanted to live. And then I found yoga.

---

[17] National Institutes of Health study on depression and aging. https://nihseniorhealth.gov/depression/aboutdepression/01.html)

"Yoga practice gave me a purpose. It also led to new friends who were more compassionate than the ones I had known. Everyone had been through something, and they weren't afraid to own it. Most of all, it helped me solidify that the world was a good place to be in, and that I wanted to stay in it. Make no mistake: Yoga saved my life."

Please do not think we are telling you to flush all your medications down the toilet and do a Downward Facing Dog because it will set you free. Not at all. You must always follow your doctor's orders. Yet practicing yoga might just help!

Long-term illness and particularly depression manifests in the body. Although the problem may be in our spirit, the body keeps the score. Depression will show up as fatigue, muscle soreness, aches and pains. According to a study in "Dialogues in Clinical Neuroscience," 69% of patients who went to the doctor for physical pain were indeed suffering from depression.[18]

The root of many a problem can be in the physical, emotional, and spiritual traumas we've endured over the years. It takes a monumental effort to do the work, to figure out what we need, and how to help ourselves. But it's worth it. Know the self, then determine what you need. An answer is waiting for you. We both know you can figure it out if you make your well-being a priority.

Midlife Yogis Have Special Needs

Older warriors are courageous, yet we need to be cautious as well to avoid pain from overdoing things. Our joints do not

---

[18] https://www.ncbi.nlm.nih.gov/pmc/articles/PMC486942/

have the same capacity for weight bearing as when we were young. Our wrists, elbows, and shoulders may have suffered from repetitive injury. Our hips and knees are cranky with overuse. Our necks are weaker. Our back may have lost suppleness. The list goes on.

Moreover, older warriors do not bounce back as quickly as those blessed with youth. So we need to weigh the risks versus the rewards of various practices and poses. Courage without caution is foolishness.

We cannot tell you for sure when you must rest and when you must get up. Only you and your physician will know. But we want to give you a guideline of things to look out for as you begin to exercise and practice yoga as an older practitioner. We are all different, but as we age we will develop similar needs.

Midlife Warriors: The Feet and Calves

Let's begin with the feet. After all, they have to support us for the rest of our lives. The foot and ankle have 26 bones, 33 joints, and more than 100 muscles, tendons and ligaments. That is a lot of opportunity for arthritis. In fact, breaking a bone in the foot is one of the most common injuries that plague us in midlife. While it is not usually life threatening, pain in the feet will almost always slow us down!

What keeps our feet young and healthy is being strong and flexible. Please follow our guidelines from Chapter One and do your stretching and strengthening exercises regularly, if not daily.

One common foot complaint is heel pain in the form of bone spurs or plantar fasciitis. The plantar fascia is a band of tough tissue connecting the heel bone to the toes. When it becomes tight or inflamed you will experience intense pain in the heel or arch of your foot.

Pain in the ball of the foot is also a typically agonizing ailment, often diagnosed as metatarsalgia. It's an inflammation generally caused by strenuous activity with improper support or ill-fitting shoes. This has also become more common among yogis lately because of overdoing a Yoga Flow or Vinyasa practice in bare feet. If you do this kind of flowing, moving yoga, be cautious about transitioning from pose to pose, and always do so, when possible, on the heel of the foot, which is meant to bear more weight than just the toes.

While the feet are a mass of tiny bones, ligaments and tendons, some of the problem actually begins just a little higher in the calves. A lifetime of walking, jogging, running, and even sitting around will tighten the calf muscle. When the calves become tight, the fascia or connective tissue will start to pull on the muscles and the bones, straining the fascia of the ankles and feet. Though painful, it can be resolved over time by stretching and strengthening.

Stretching the Calves:

Massage

Start with massage. If using your hands is not enough, we recommend utilizing little balls such as the Radroller™ or Therapy Balls. These can be found on the internet.

Calf Smashing

Calf smashing is an Iyengar Yoga technique designed to release the fascia of the calves. Kneel on the floor and place a rolled up mat, or small towel rolled tightly, across the center of both calves. Then sit back on it. Each time apply as much pressure as you can bear. To make it harder and more effective, use a harder object. A wooden rolling pin brings great results. Remember to breathe!

Ankle Stretching

The three specific ankle joints move in all four directions: forward and back, and side-to-side. However, our ankles easily lose flexibility and strength, becoming vulnerable to strains or breaks. Garland Pose, *Malasana*, is the ankle fixer-upper. With the inner edges of the feet together, widen your knees to the side and squat deeply, stretching your ankles to the side and the heels to the floor. Stretching the arms out in front will also help release the lower back. Another variation would be to stand with feet hip distance apart and squat into a little ball.

Strengthening the Ankle and Calf

Strengthening the ankles and calves happens naturally as we walk and move, yet we can also make them stronger with focused exercise. Calf raises are the best. Stand with both feet on a block or a stair. Slowly lift yourself up and down. Then try to balance on one leg at a time. Use all parts of the foot, toes, arch and calf. For the ankles, repeat this exercise with the heels together and the feet turned out, and then the opposite way, with toes together and heels turned out.

Midlife Warriors: The Knees and Hips

Our joints usually give us some trouble in midlife. Reasons for that vary, yet the most common are overuse and poor posture. Our human species has evolved over the past hundred years into spending time in chairs rather than standing and moving about. We are no longer hunters and gatherers, but drivers and sitters.

Joints and cartilage simply wear out with time. Knee replacement is the number one joint surgery for older Americans. According to a National Hospital Discharge Survey, between the years 2000 and 2010, more than 5.2 million total knee replacements were performed in the United States. By 2010, the operation had become the leading inpatient surgery for adults aged 45 or older. Hip replacements are not far behind. During those same years, the number of annual procedures more than doubled, from 138,700 in 2000 to 310,800 in 2010, according to a report in HealthDay.

Interestingly, hip replacements were once the domain of those 75 and older, but now are being performed much earlier on those aged 45 or older. What's going on? For one thing, our generation of midlife warriors has been the most active of all generations. Because we exercise frequently and have come to enjoy a vigorous lifestyle, our activities put stress on our joints. And we have not been very good at slowing down.

We don't have to actually slow down, but we do have to take care of our knees and hips. If we maintain strength and flexibility in our joints, we'll be able to enjoy an active lifestyle for longer than what many people think is possible.

The Delicate Knees

First off, do not argue with your knees. It is like arguing with a toddler; you won't win. There is no pushing through pain or working through a nagging twinge in the knee joint. Discomfort is a sign that you must cease and desist. Furthermore, a "pop" is a sign that it's game over, time to see a surgeon.

Knees do not move sideways; they only hinge forward and back. A quick, sharp twist can bring about misery and pain. Twisting is the job of the hips, which should be able to move in four directions. However, if the hips are tight and cannot open from side to side, or front to back, then undue pressure is placed on the knees. Indeed, the best knee exercises would be to create mobility and strength in the hips. However, there are things we can do to keep the knees happy and strong starting with alignment.

In any yoga pose or physical activity, you must make sure your knees are properly aligned. In standing poses always make sure the knee appears straight. When doing a lunge, make sure the knee is positioned over the ankle so the shin can help support your weight and your strong hamstrings support the body. The tendons are not meant to hold a 175-pound person. That's the job of the bones and muscles. And yet if you do a standing lunge, or worse, balance on one bent leg with all your weight in front of the ankle, then that's exactly what you're asking the knee ligaments to do. The center of the knee should also appear to be lined up with the second toe. You can do this by simply taking a visual before you move into a position.

In seated poses, make sure there is no knee pain. The calf supports the knee. Engage your feet and legs to support the knee. You can engage the shin by flexing your feet, particularly the pinky toes. Start by sitting on a block or a bolster. If you are sitting in "easy pose," or "crisscross applesauce," then flex your feet to protect your knees. If you are sitting with your feet tucked behind you, notice if your foot and knee appear straight. During any exercise work your feet and the arches strongly, and make sure they are aligned to support the knees.

Hero's Pose, *Supta Virasana*

Like many things in life, Hero's Pose can be a blessing or a curse. Achieved correctly, it's a good way to reinstate blood flow to the joints and surrounding tissue. Yet done incorrectly it can deprive the delicate tissue of nourishment and tweak the tendons. Sit on a block, bolster, or on the floor with your legs folded behind you. Engage your feet by pressing all ten toenails firmly into the ground. If you have any pain in the knee, you must elevate your seat until the discomfort is relieved, or move out of the pose. Hold the position for 20 to 30 seconds. Then straighten out your legs immediately. The benefit of the pose is to promote circulation to the joint. However, research indicates that too much time in this pose can cause irreversible damage to the delicate tissue. How much is too much? Listen to your knees. They will tell you.

Back of the Knee Pressure

Similar to Calf Smashing, it is useful to apply pressure in the form of a ball, a rolled up yoga mat, or a small hard tube to the back of the knee. Sit on your heels or feet for approximately thirty seconds to a minute. Then immediately straighten your legs, flooding the joint with fresh blood and loosening the fascia behind it.

Midlife Warriors: Maintaining the Hips

As we age, work, sit, and just go through the motions of life, our hips will naturally lose both strength and mobility. Then the need to move in all four directions is usually delegated to the knee, and that is not its job. Arthritis, the loss of cartilage, tightness and even weakness are common complaints among those with poorly performing hips, greatly impacting our mobility.

Strengthening the Hips:

Triangle Pose, *Trikonasana*

Triangle Pose is a stretch and a strengthener all in one. Take a wide stance by extending your arms out to the side and placing your ankles beneath your wrists. Point your front foot forwards. Shorten your feet, engage your legs and squeeze your feet and shins into the midline. Using the strength from your inner thighs, push your groins and sitting bones back and apart. Put your corset to work and squeeze your glutes as you slide your hand down your front leg slowly and steadily.

Tabletop Leg Lifts

In Tabletop position, with your hands and knees on the floor, slowly lift one leg at a time. Keeping your hips level, lift and lower a straight leg to the back, then to the side, building strength as you go. Repeat with the leg bent, as in the old-fashioned "fire hydrant" exercises.

Stretching the Hips:

Half Pigeon Pose, *Eka Pada Rajakapotasana*

Half Pigeon Pose is an excellent stretch for the outer hips. Always keep your calves and feet engaged and squeeze them toward the midline. Move your sitting bones back and apart with your strong inner thighs. Keep your corset very strong as you bend toward the ground. If this pose causes pain in the knee, you can also do it on your back in a "Figure Four" variation.

Cowface Pose, *Gomukhasana*

For stretching the outer hips, take a Tabletop Pose with hands and knees on the mat, place one knee behind the other. Slowly lower your hips to the ground. We will pray for you.

Seated Wide Angle Pose, *Upavistha Konasana*

For the inner thighs, sit on your mat or a block with legs apart. With strongly flexed feet and engaged leg muscles, squeeze your feet and shins into the midline and then move your sitting bones back and apart. Reach back with your hand and feel for a pronounced lumbar curve. Sit on a blanket to keep your lumbar curve even when sitting straight. Once you can do that and straighten your legs, it is safe to bend forward or to the side. Always keep your corset strength and avoid bending forward in this pose if you cannot sit in front of your sitting bones, as it will hurt your back.

Supine Frog Pose

From Tabletop Pose, slowly widen the knees keeping the core engaged, stretching the inner thighs and hips. Hold for 20 seconds or more.

Low Lunge Pose or *Anjaneyasana* Stretches

For the front and back of hips, take a Lunge Pose, then lower the back knee to the ground. Keeping the groin in a neutral pelvis position and the core strong, slowly lower the quad of the back leg to the floor. Then reverse the pose to Runner's Lunge extending the hips back.

Midlife Warriors: The Back

We are only as young as our back is supple, and strong. Today it seems "normal" to live with back pain; it is the number one cause of chronic pain for all adults. According to the American Chiropractic Association, 80% of us will experience back pain in our lives.

Nourishing the spine, while keeping it strong and supple should be our number one priority for a physical yoga practice. Pain in this area causes most of our problems! Yet by far, the back is the area that often gives us a source of constant mystery. "What did I do to my back?" we might ask. Here are a few more interesting facts about back pain from the American Chiropractic Association:

Back Pain Facts

- *Low back pain is the leading cause of disability worldwide.*

- *Back pain is outnumbered only by the common cold for why people see a doctor.*

- *Most causes are due to postural misalignment and not a serious condition such as arthritis, infection, fracture, or cancer.*

- *Americans spend at least $50 billion each year on back pain.*

Often it is back pain that brings people to yoga for the first time.

Strengthening the Back:

Bridge Pose, *Setu Bandhasana*

Lie on your back with the soles of the feet on the floor, hip distance apart. Keeping your head, shoulders and hips on the floor, lift your hips up without tucking your tail. Squeeze your feet and shins toward the midline and skillfully lower your pelvis to maintain the lumbar curve. Continue squeezing the bottom tips of your shoulder blades toward each other. Press your upper arms into the floor in order to help lift the back of your heart with the tips of your shoulder blades. Breathing steadily, move your hips toward the floor and your heart toward your head so that you are extending your spine in two directions simultaneously.

Rabbit Pose, *Sasangasana*

Sitting on your heels, reach back and hold the outer ankles. Tuck your chin to your chest and pull your core back in toward your spine. Try to touch your forehead to the top of the knees. Then slide your head to the floor. With no weight in the head, pull your core back and up until the thighs are vertical. If you have any weakness in the neck, then place your hands on the floor by the knees, keep your head above the floor, and perform a very strong "Halloween Cat" move. Make sure the muscles of the back and core are firing.

Plank Pose

Place your hands on the floor beneath your shoulders and extend your feet back until the body is straight. Squeeze your feet and legs toward the midline and create a small lumbar curve. Pull up your lower abs and rib anchor for support. Squeeze arms toward the midline and keep your head level. Hold for 30 seconds and work up to a minute.

Locust Pose, *Salabhasana*

Lying on your belly, with arms outstretched in a T-shape, begin by lifting the torso and legs off the floor. Hold for 20 seconds or five breaths. Be sure to use your lower abdominal core or "rib anchor" strength. It will save your back.

Stretching the Back

The spine can stretch in six directions: Forward and back, side to side, and twisting around. It's important to do all these variations daily to keep the spine supple.

Side-to-Side Stretching, *Indudalasana*

Standing in Mountain Pose, reach the arms overhead and clasp the hands or hold a strap. Keep the hips steady and facing forward while gently stretching to the right. Hold for 20 seconds; then stretch to the left. You can also place the side of your hip, right and left, against a wall to increase the stretch and for steadiness. A more accessible stretch would be to take Child's Pose and walk the arms side to side, keeping the hips steady.

Forward and Backward Cat and Cow Stretch

In Tabletop Pose, with hands and knees on a mat, look up and allow your back to sag like a happy, heavy cow. Then take the opposite shape and round your spine like a Halloween cat. This is one of the simplest, yet most efficient ways to build a supple spine.

Twisted Lunge, *Parivrtta Parsvakonasana*

Step forward into Lunge Pose, then bring the back knee down to the mat. Keep your legs steady by hugging to the midline, then bring your hands together in prayer and lean toward the front leg. Press your elbow against your leg to get some leverage while twisting. A more accessible version is to sit in a chair. Keeping the knees together, twist to one side. Remember never force a stretch.

Backward Bending

Contrary to the belief that bending backwards is dangerous, it is actually quite healing if done correctly. All the work of the feet, legs, and core apply even though you are bending backwards. A beginning backbend approach would be to lie on the floor and place a block in the stiffest part of your upper back, and another block under your head. Maintain for 30 seconds, working up to a minute or more.

Midlife Warriors: The Upper Body

The neck and shoulders are actually the third largest source of chronic pain in adults, according to the American Osteopathic Association. If you think about it, remember the head is an 11-pound bowling ball balanced precariously on seven little cervical bones. If you've ever been suddenly jarred in motion, as in an accident, then that head can feel like 60 pounds when bouncing back and forth. In addition, those tiny bones and joints wear out over time, yet they still must support the head.

Then take into account our penchant for extreme sports such as heli-skiing and bungee jumping. Even the activities we did as kids, perhaps football, soccer or ice skating, often contribute to long-term injury. Extreme sports are responsible for 40,000 head and neck injuries a year, according to a study performed by the Western Michigan University School of Medicine in Kalamazoo.[19] "While we've been inventing all these new sports, the conversation has been all about the excitement and not about the safety," said study co-author Dr. Vani Sabesan, an assistant professor in the department of orthopedic surgery.

However, you don't have to be participating in the Olympics to break a bone. Michelle fractured four cervical

---

[19] Vani J. Sabesan, MD, presented to the American Academy of Orthopedic Surgeons, March 2014.

vertebrae while sleeping on a plane. "You know how your head sometimes bobs back and forth?" she remembers. "Well, mine bobbed backwards and I felt a stabbing pain like none other."

For most of us, like Michelle, the neck needs to be strengthened.

"I often see the neck as a place we forget to exercise," Desiree points out. "With five major muscle groups, our neck needs to stay strong just like every other part of our body."

The shoulders also have special needs. Poor posture, lax core muscles, injury, and illness will contribute to shoulder problems as we age. We may develop tendinitis, bursitis, acute arthritis, losing mobility, flexibility, and strength.

Shoulders are particularly delicate since they are the most hypermobile part of our anatomy. If you look more closely at your upper body, the arm bone is connected to the torso by an interconnected web of muscle and tendon called the "rotator cuff." If any part of this fragile bionetwork is out of alignment, it will place stress on another set of muscles. Then, like a worn spot in a piece of fabric, that place will give way if it is stressed.

When the neck has become weak, and if we have developed a rounded posture in the head, neck and upper back, that will also damage our shoulder girdle. Then the shoulders will round forward, creating both a weakness in the front and an over-stretching in the back. Yoga practice can correct this imbalance through a more aligned and strengthened posture.

If you have an injury to your neck or spinal cord, please consult your physician before starting any exercise program. This part of your body is not to be messed with. However, we as yoga teachers and long-time practitioners feel that to maintain life with a minimal amount of pain, it is crucial to focus our attention on strengthening certain injury-prone areas.

Stretching the Neck

- Stand with your back against a wall. Keeping your head and shoulders on the wall, slowly turn your head side to side. Remember not to ever force any movement regarding your head and neck.

- Lie on your back, knees bent, with the soles of the feet on the floor. Make sure your shoulders are in alignment with the shoulder blades on your back. Turn your head gently side to side.

Words of Caution

One thing we ask you to be cautious about is stretching the neck forwards and backwards. As a society, we are chronically over-stretching the neck forward to view a computer screen, read text messages on a phone, and/or drive a car. This tendency to stretch forward has created a laxness in our neck muscles sometimes called "text neck." Likewise, most of us stretch the neck backwards incorrectly by throwing it back. When looking up and back, be sure to maintain your neck strength by keeping your chin pointed down, as if you are holding a large orange to your chest. We describe this further at the end of the chapter. When you are stretching, use all the supporting muscles of the neck, upper shoulders and core to bend and do not ever throw the head back mindlessly.

Strengthening the Neck

- Lie with your back on the floor and extend your skull as if you are attempting to make your neck longer. You should be working so intensely that your head feels heavy. Try to barely lift your head off the floor about ¼ inch. Hold for 10 to 30 seconds. This is much harder than it looks.

- Lie with your belly on the floor. Cross your arms and place your forehead on them. Gently press your head into your forearms and hold for 10 seconds. Increase to 30 seconds.

- Sitting in a chair, place one hand behind your head. With your chin slightly tucked, press your head back into your hand. Hold for 10 seconds. Increase to 30 seconds.

- Stand with your back on a wall. With your chin slightly tucked, press your head up and back, as if you were trying to be taller and place more of your cervical spine on the wall. Press and release for 10 to 20 seconds at a time.

- Practice Bridge Pose by lying on your back with the soles of the feet flat on the floor. Isometrically draw your feet back toward your hips. With arms by your sides, elevate your hips and chest into the air. Press your head down as much as you can, which will strengthen your neck.

Stretching the Shoulders

- Stand in the center of your mat and hold a strap out in front with your hands shoulder width apart. Lift the strap up over your head and bend your arms. Take the belt back slowly to stretch your inner shoulders and pectoral muscles.

- Stand with your shoulder next to the wall, and place your arm alongside the wall behind you. Press the front of the shoulder into the wall as you slowly turn your torso into the center of the room.

- Lie belly down with your arms out in a T-shape. Slowly roll over onto one arm, bending the top leg to support your weight. Repeat on both sides.

- Stand in the center of your mat and clasp both hands behind you. If you cannot reach your other hand, use a strap or towel to make the connection. Slowly pull the arms back, while maintaining your core strength. If you're able, bend forward and allow the hands to come up over your head.

- Stand and hold a yoga belt behind you in both hands. Squeeze the bottom of your shoulder blades toward each other and lift your heart. Widen your stance and bend over allowing your arms to come down toward the floor.

Strengthening the Shoulders

Once we start to open the front of the shoulders, then we need to continue to strengthen the shoulder girdle.

Standing Arm Rotations

Stand tall and extend the arms wide. Squeeze the arms so the muscles are fully engaged. Rotate your arms so the palms face front, down and back. Do this several times to develop strength and flexibility.

Side Plank Pose, *Vasisthasana*

From Downward Facing Dog, place one hand in the center of the mat. Roll your hips and heels to the side and lift your top arm. Maintain your shoulder blade on the back and utilize strong core support. You can lower the bottom leg to your knee for stability, or come to your forearm if needed.

Midlife Warriors: The Wrists

Unfortunately, there has been an abundance of wrist injuries among yogis of all ages. This is particularly nagging for older yogis, as the wrist easily suffers from repetitive use. Working on a computer, using hand tools, peeling potatoes, gardening, knitting, and such all contribute to injury. However, specifically in yoga, misalignment in a pose and neglecting to engage our larger core muscles are usually the culprits behind wrist pain.

When practicing yoga, refrain from putting excessive weight on your wrists. Do not ever place weight on the base of the palm for an extended period of time, particularly in

Downward Facing Dog or Cobra Pose. If you can easily lift your fingers in these poses, then there is too much tension and weight on the back of your hand. Be sure to press the thumb and pointer fingers into the mat and keep the weight on the ridges of your hands where the fingers meet the palm. Maintain a tiny bit of space under your palm and where the wrist meets the floor so that a ladybug or a paper clip could fit in there.

Strengthening the Wrists

In Downward Facing Dog, or Tabletop position lift up the back of your hands so your weight is resting on the ridges and fingers. Then slowly lower to the ground in a kind of "wrist push-up." For more of a challenge, put your hands on a block with the wrists and thumbs stretching off the front.

Stretching the Wrists

- To begin, massage the front and back of your wrist. Then extend your arm in front of your body with the palm face up. Stretch your wrists down toward the floor, keeping the fingers straight, not bent. Then repeat the stretch one finger at a time. Turn the hand over and repeat the stretch in the opposite direction.

- In Tabletop, place the hands on the floor, then reverse them so the fingers are pointing toward the knees. Gently move forward and back to stretch your wrists.

- In Gorilla, or stand in *Uttanasana*, fold over as if you are touching your toes, and place the palms under your feet. Move the feet up to the wrists to stretch them out.

Do Not Give Up!

Pain, injury and illness are natural consequences of being alive. We grow, we stumble, and we start again. These setbacks serve to slow us down and also wake us up. They are the gift, if you will, of leading full and active lives. It is easy to forget that we are human and not superhuman; an injury helps us remember to put ourselves and our well-being in first place.

Life is about balance. Learning to make our health a priority is often the teaching. There may be days where it's all we can do to just get out of bed. The idea of practice may be a monumental effort. But it is not the big things that we must do at these times. It is the smallest of things. That is the path to wellness.

Yoga is not a single practice. Yoga is a lifetime of being attuned to the body, mind, and spirit. It is being alert. There are the big showy poses, and then there are the smallest of actions that produce the grandest of results. When life slows us down, practice, even if it is just to sit and breathe.

Pain creates awareness. And awareness is yoga.
Pain creates patience. Be patient with yourself.
Pain makes us pay attention to tension.

Remember, if it hurts, it's not yoga. Causing ourselves pain is not yoga. In many ways, practicing with moderation is the most yogic perspective. Pain may be our opportunity to invite real change in our lives that will make us stronger for years to come.

Slowing down is not for sissies. It's for those who wish to create long-lasting transformation, and who will never, ever give up their right to a healthy and strong life.

The Practice:
Warrior Heal Thy Neck!

New technology means we spend more time with our heads in forward and downward positions looking at screens. This takes its toll on the neck. Certainly cavemen did not have these problems.

Strengthening

- Try to do the strengthening exercises we mentioned earlier, at least once a day.

Stretching

- Be very careful when extending the neck. Even though it may feel good to pull hard and stretch your neck side to side or bring the ear to the shoulder, that kind of aggressive stretching actually makes your neck tighter and more protective. You may use your hand to gently stretch but you want to resist isometrically. An intense stretching sensation may actually cause more harm than good.

- Sitting in an easy, cross-legged position, gently place one hand on the side of your head and press to one side, resisting the stretch the entire time. Repeat on the other; then gently press forward. To stretch backward, keep your neck muscles engaged by moving the sides of the throat back as if to make a double chin. Then stretch back. This maintains a proper cervical alignment.

Yoga Poses to Strengthen the Neck

Strengthen our necks to keep our head on straight!

Bridge Pose, *Setu Bandhasana*
Lie on the floor, with feet parallel on the mat. Try to bring the feet close to the trunk so they either touch the hips, or so that you can graze the feet with your fingertips. Bring your hands by your sides, bend at the elbow and face the hands inward, like a robot's arms. Press the arms down and lift the chest. Eventually you will be able to also lift the hips. Gently press the back of the head into the mat, holding for a few seconds each time.

Camel, *Ustrasana*, with "Double Chin Face"
Kneeling with your toes tucked under, squeeze your feet and shins to the midline. Take your thighs back to create a lumbar curve and then engage your corset. Squeeze the bottom tips of your shoulder blades toward each other and lift your heart. Stretch your spine in two directions, from underneath your ribcage, out through the tailbone and up through your neck and head. Keeping the sides of

your throat back will greatly strengthen your neck. If you are very strong and you want to take your head back make sure it is your neck taking your head back with strength rather than your head falling back like a whiplash. The head moves with the neck as if to make a double chin, so you always keep your head in a strong line of energy.

Grace	Pose	Grit
Kneeling, working the neck	Camel	Hands at heels, full backbend
Lying supine, chest lifted	Bridge Pose	Hands grip ankles, hips lift

Prevention is the best medicine.
To see a video tutorial of these poses, go to
www.YogaDownload.com

Fearless After Fifty: Practical Advice
Heal Thyself

Easy and inexpensive

- Take a nap, or a 10-minute Savasana.

- Designate a time for healing rituals such as baths, soothing oils, massage, or reading.

- Ask a teacher to show you how to do a pose correctly.

- Try supplements and oils.

- Make nutritional smoothies and drink your greens.

More ... money, time and focus
- Maybe it's time for a spa day!

- Try acupuncture and cupping therapies.

- A therapeutic massage targets the deeper, underlying muscles and fascia.

All in!
- Consult a doctor if you are in pain. Don't give up.

- Strengthen your core with Pilates classes.

- Try Physical Therapy for long-term chronic injury and pain relief.

- Commit to a series of private yoga sessions to experience one-on-one alignment.

- Hire a Personal Trainer to make sure you are exercising right.

Seven
Equanimity and Balance

The secret to having it all is loving it all.
~ Dr. Joyce Brothers

Before we get your hopes up too much that there is such a thing as balance, let us set the record straight: It ain't gonna happen. Balance is more of a fairy tale than a true state of being.

Balance in life is elusive. This thing we seek—this moment of perfect clarity and harmony—is like a Ping-Pong ball traveling from one side of the table to the other. Balance is the moment in the middle. We like to imagine it in slow motion, just frame by frame going o-v-e-r t-h-e n-e-t. Good luck holding onto it. Why would we even try?

Elizabeth Gilbert explains, "To say that someone has found the secret to a balanced life is to suggest that they have solved life, and that they now float through their days in a constant state of grace and ease, never suffering stress, ambivalence, confusion, exhaustion, anger, fear, or regret. Which is a wonderful description of nobody, ever."

Balance is fleeting; the Universe gives us just enough of it so that we want more. The balance between work and play, family and friends, taking care of an older generation and/or mothering a younger one, individual needs versus the needs of our community—all of it is more of a wild ride than an end result.

Trying to stay in this unrealistic place of the middle puts a huge burden on us. Are we supposed to be calm? Find that perfect state? Be an eye that doesn't blink in the storm?

Midlife could be the most out of balance time of all. Just when we are supposed to have our act together, we are sandwiched by older relatives who need love and care, and younger children who still need support. Some of us may have grandchildren who need childcare. We may have health and financial issues, while some of us may be stressed about retirement. Others may go back to work due to shrinking reserves and a desire to be useful. Some of us are running businesses; some of us may feel that a business is running us.

Do we need more time to get it all done? Or would more time mean we'd be doing *more*? What if instead, we focused on loving our life?

Pleasure May Be the Point

We asked Judith Hanson Lasater, PhD, PT, the founder of *Yoga Journal* and longtime yogi and Iyengar instructor, how is it that she thrives in today's world? "I try to squeeze as much pleasure as I can, out of every single moment."

Simple, yes? Easy, no! Remember, if we lived "a problem-free life," then no matter what was happening in our lives, we could find a way to enjoy it. It's the difference between "having" to do something and "getting" to do something.

"Pleasure causes the most wonderful cascade of biochemical hormones and changes in your body that are healthy to you," said Judith. "I say yes to pleasure every chance I can. For me it's my practice, my bath, having the foods I love. It's enjoying something fully.

"The things that give me pleasure and joy I want to make sure are in my life every day. I spend time cultivating, choosing and valuing them. The joy I feel to have people over for dinner. Setting the table beautifully. My favorite hand creams. It's really very simple things that I try to find every day, and I make sure there is some joy."

Balance is Bliss

Interestingly, the people we know who are the busiest and the most out of balance, are not necessarily the unhappiest. In fact, in our extremely unscientific, undocumented and unproven study of friends and family, it seems that the correlation between being chaotic and being unhappy, isn't necessarily related.

Apparently, you can be over-scheduled and over-tired and still be ecstatic about your life (Michelle!). You can travel every weekend, babysit for your granddaughter during the week, move, plan retreats, write a book, and still find time to squeeze in joy (Desiree!) Or you could be perfectly in balance, have not that much to do, and be a bit blah (people we won't name). Really, we know individuals like that.

There's no explaining to a person who claims to be really busy, what busy is, when they don't have a job, or go to school, or have children at home, or have a parent to care for, or have anything whatsoever on their calendar. If a person thinks they are terribly busy, then they are going to be terribly busy.

Then it naturally follows that if you think you are having it all, and loving every minute, then you absolutely are doing just that.

The way to feeling balanced in life begins by taking stock of where you are, and what you need. We know that a peaceful, sensible, well-adjusted state of being exists, and we can squeeze every bit of pleasure out of it even if only for short periods of time. It is comforting to know that calm is as close as a five-minute meditation. We can also appreciate every second of a *Savasana* at the end of our yoga practice. We know that a day will end with a restorative evening ritual of a bath and a good book.

Knowing that this peaceful, balanced state exists allows us to dedicate ourselves fully to keeping up with the craziness of a life well lived. A moment of pure bliss is as close as a piece of chocolate. You just have to enjoy the bajeezus out of it!

Calm Is Closer Than You Think

If we are seeking ways to feel more in balance, it helps to know what exactly it is that we want. Is it stability? Is it joy? Is it a sense of purpose? Is it to feel useful? Is it more money? Is it more time? Is it more love?

The way to coping when life is very much out of control is to go inside of yourself and see what you need to feel whole again. We know that you know what you want. Nobody else can answer that for you. Only you. One person may have a deep desire to feel relevant again. Another may wish to serve or volunteer to feel useful. Someone else may need 10 minutes of absolute peace and quiet to get their act together. No matter what you need, you are closer than you think to having it all.

Take Five Minutes and Answer These Questions

1. *What specific use of your time is making you unhappy?*
2. *What activity would you rather be doing?*
3. *What would you like to cultivate? Relevance? Usefulness? Harmony?*
4. *What is one tiny thing you can do to achieve this?*
5. *Can you make your well-being your conscious priority?*
6. *Can you support this decision on a daily basis?*

It's the Little Things

Figuring out what you need is the first rung to getting it. Then find the *smallest* solution to take the next, tiniest step. Big changes are made of little steps, not the other way around.

You see, as human beings we strive to find world peace, or feed every child on the planet, and yet we cannot get our own dinner on the table. We want to be Mother Teresa, but in reality we can barely keep up with being Mother Desiree or Mother Michelle. So instead of looking at the big picture of your lifespan over 100 years, try to focus on the most minuscule change you can make in a single day.

Small changes are manageable. You can see them. You can imagine them. You can try them on. And if they don't work, nothing major is sacrificed.

Yoga teaches us that it's the incremental changes that get us into the pose, and not the other way around. We might think, "Oh we want to master a Handstand." So we spend our time jumping upside down unsuccessfully, over and over. Like Albert Einstein's definition of insanity: Why are you doing the same thing over and over again, and expecting different results?

Instead, what is the smallest thing you can do? To get to a Handstand, can you set your hands on the floor with intention? Then try to work your finger pads to grip? Can you engage your arms? Can you stretch and extend your legs just a little more? Are you able to strengthen your core and engage the abdominal lock? Can you keep your kicking leg straight? By focusing on these little itty bitty things, you will see a change in your practice. Then one day, poof, you get the pose.

If you are seeking more balance in your life, ask yourself what is literally the least you can do.

Baby Steps for Balance

- **If you need a breather …**
  Can you make yourself a cup of tea every afternoon? Just 15 minutes may revive you.

- **If your mind is racing …**
  Can you sit quietly for just five minutes? Five minutes actually works.

- **If you need more exercise …**
  Can you wake up just 20 minutes earlier? Or take the stairs at work? Or take a walk at lunch?

- **If you need more human connection …**
  Can you volunteer just one afternoon a week doing something you love?

- **If you need help with childcare …**
  Can you enlist the help of a neighbor? Or inquire what options exist at your local community center?

- **If you need more love …**
  Can you adopt a pet, volunteer at a shelter, or get a goldfish?

- **If you are lonely …**
  Can you ask just one person you know to join you for a movie or tea? Just one?

- **If your home is a mess …**
  Can you make just one night a week housework time?

Lame Excuses Are Lame

We know that some of you read that list of suggestions and realize, "Oh wow. Change is easier than I thought." And we also know that some of you read that list and itemized a dozen reasons why nothing will work to help you out of your rut. We know this, because we know people like you.

When confronted with change, every one of us will make lame excuses from time to time. We say things like, "Oh I can't do that," or "That is not me." Is this the truth? Or is this resistance piping up?

Remember, our minds do not like change. The mind is controlled by ego, which is a fearful, quaking mass of matter. The mind is not naturally our best friend, or our most supportive teacher. It is like the mother-in-law who tells you that you can never be good enough for her child. The mind is a "meddle-in-law"! It doesn't care if you're miserable. Its entire purpose is to keep things exactly as they are because it dreads change of any kind. So thank it for sharing and move forward.

Here is the truth: The tiniest change you make will bring you that much closer to a sense of balance. Literally, we want you to think of the very least thing you can do. Remember, no effort is ever wasted. You will have more time to experience pure pleasure, and enjoy all the rest of it as well. What's more, now you have a path back to calm precisely when you need it the most.

For instance, you will not *die* of sleep deprivation from just sleeping 20 minutes less a day. It's true. Death by sleep deprivation takes about 115 hours or between 11 and 19 days of nonstop activity. We looked it up! Furthermore, if you incorporate exercise into your life, you may find that your quality of sleep is better overall, so you need less.

You will not be utterly devastated if you miss just one night of your favorite television show to clean the house. That is why someone invented recording devices. You will not be the worst parent if you get help or find a sitter one afternoon a week. In fact, you may be better for it and your kids will get a taste of independence. All of this whacky thinking that keeps us stuck comes from our ego.

What we need is the mind making less creative excuses and contributing to more creative thinking. Often our lack of equanimity stems from a lack of imaginative solutions. The first step is to understand what we need. Then look for the tiniest, least possible, most unobtrusive way to begin. Baby steps will get us to a place of balance.

"The journey of a thousand miles begins with a single step," Confucius said.

Once you find the smallest, simplest, least complicated first step, then it's up to you to make it happen. It's not up to your family. It's not up to your co-workers. It's not up to the Universe! It's only up to you.

We are not asking you to make a huge transformation in your life. We are asking that you try the tiniest adjustment. Trying things on is the only way to see if they fit. Go for a little modification, or a sense of being okay, and leave discovering paradise for another day.

"I am giving up on this idea of finding bliss," declares Christina Sell, who teaches yoga worldwide. Bliss is big. It's *Samadhi* or full-on enlightenment. It's also unfathomable to many individuals who live in the real world. "I am searching instead for a deep sense of okay-ness," Christina said.

Go for "okay-ness." Relish moments of pleasure. Realize you get to do this, and not that you have to. Take a baby step toward balance and you might find that rather than seeking the whole enchilada of enlightenment, you are happy with a smaller morsel once a day.

The Power of Rituals

Establishing supportive rituals might be the answer to seeking balance in our day. Deepak Chopra, MD, a longtime yoga practitioner, explains that establishing a positive daily ritual is "perpetually transformative." He tells us, "As adults in an over-stimulated and stressful world, it's difficult to create habits like this. We feel powerless to control what's going on in our heads much less stay focused and disciplined enough to make big life changes. As a result, we've lost touch with our inherent power to heal, grow, and manifest our fullest potential. And despite all the material abundance in our lives, we suffer."

"The best way to quiet the mind and unlock your inner power is to start small when creating new daily rituals,"

Chopra continues. "Through the ancient teachings of yoga, we know that our thoughts lead to actions; our actions become habits; our habits form our character; and our character determines our destiny. Daily ritual is the act of taking positive thoughts and putting them into action."

Desiree's rituals begin with honoring her body so she can take care of her mind and spirit. She makes a point of drinking copious amounts of water, especially with lemon. Other personal routines include dry brushing her skin and performing facial "yoga exercises" as a muscle toner. "It's better than Botox™!" she quips.

Morning exercise is also one of Desiree's rituals, either in the form of a walk, practicing yoga, or weight lifting. She has been taking care of herself in this way for decades, even when her children were very young. "If I honor my bodily temple by hydrating and moving it every day, it makes me more productive. I prefer to practice or work out alone in the mornings, as that is also my meditation time. I find these rituals heighten my creativity."

Desiree's evening ritual includes expressing gratitude for every person and each blessing in her life. This practice is soothing to her mind, helping her fall asleep more peacefully.

Michelle starts every single day with a ritual of enjoying a cup of tea and sitting quietly. She may meditate, or read, or write in a journal, but absolutely she starts with tea. When she travels, she brings her kettle, tea, and cup with her. She makes this quiet time happen, no matter what else is scheduled for the day. "Sometimes my life feels so busy, so overwhelming, that I wake up and know at least I have this time with my tea, looking out my window, writing in a journal, and sitting calmly.

It's absolutely double-dog guaranteed in a world where nothing is really certain."

Michelle also prefers to bathe rather than shower, making it a special time to relax. She honors her body with fragrant oils and a Korean scrubbing cloth, with plenty of replenishing masks for her face and hair. We know there are busy days that cannot accommodate the preparation, soaking and peaceful qualities of a bath versus the quick and efficient use of a shower. However, being efficient is not the point for her. "A bath is part of my daily ritual," Michelle said. "Having these set practices gives me a time and place for quiet appreciation and gratitude. A friend once told me a bath takes too much time, and I said, 'Yes, that's exactly the point.'"

Creating and performing daily rituals is putting you at the top of your priority list. It's like saying you matter. It's making the commitment to your own well-being, in the smallest and easiest way possible.

"Once a positive ritual takes hold in your life, you don't even need to think about it," Chopra wrote. "Just like brushing your teeth—it simply happens."

The Ritual of Sleep

One natural consequence of living a busy and rewarding life is that we often don't get enough sleep. What's more, aging often comes with changes to our sleep patterns. Therefore, midlife becomes a time to pay more attention to how we prepare for bed so that we can sleep more deeply if possible.

Every year it may become harder to fall asleep and stay asleep, yet it is a common misconception that as we age we need less sleep. Normal adults of any age still need six to eight hours of deep rest, according to the National Sleep Foundation.

What is messing us up? In certain cases, snoring or sleep apnea will keep us awake or interrupt the amount of oxygen we take in as the muscles in the back of our throat become lax. Hormonal changes in menopause, and even "man"-opause, will also disrupt our sleep. The amount of light we are exposed to, and our exercise routine also affects our sleep habit patterns. And lastly, alcohol has been shown to be a sleep disrupter as the sugars first make us drowsy, but then later on wake us up with an energy burst.

One of the most powerful women in the world, Arianna Huffington, analyzed the need for sleep in her book, *The Sleep Revolution*. "I studied, I met with medical doctors, scientists, and I'm here to tell you that the way to a more productive, more inspired, more joyful life is getting enough sleep," she asserts.

Technology is also proven to disrupt our sleep. "The light from our devices is short-wavelength-enriched, meaning it has a higher concentration of blue light than natural light—and blue light affects levels of the sleep-inducing hormone melatonin more than any other wavelength," according to author Jessica Schmerler.[20]

So what can we do? Turn off your phones, tablets, and computers at night! That is a start. Don't even keep them near your bed if you don't want to be disturbed. Then establish an evening ritual designed to promote a calm, serene sleep. You have to make each evening something that is expected and

---

[20] Jessica Schmerler, *Scientific American*, "The Truth About Blue Light, Sleep and Health," Sept 1, 2015.

predictable. What throws the body off is too much excitement before bed.

If you have trouble sleeping, try a practice of meditation, or a bit of gentle, peaceful stretching. You can also listen to a yoga meditation or visualization designed to relax your body. Whatever you choose, do it as a ritual for at least an hour before bed. Keep your bedtime and waking time consistent as much as possible.

Further, if you take an afternoon nap, limit its length to 20 minutes so you can still go to sleep at your normal bedtime. If you find that you are waking up very early, and also sleeping for several hours in the afternoon and going to bed quite late, then you need to alter your schedule. There is nothing more restorative for the body than eight hours of uninterrupted quality sleep during the night.

This Is Your Time

Chances are by the time you have reached midlife, you've had a job and taken responsibility for everyone and everything. Now it's time to make your own well-being a conscious priority.

Robert Holden, PhD, the creator of the blog, *Shift Happens*, explains that if you are seeking balance and had 10% more time to your day, the question isn't what *more* would you do? It's what would you do less?

Self-neglect, Dr. Holden says, is one of the leading ways we limit our sense of happiness and balance. The irony is we don't take those few minutes for ourselves because we think we're doing others a favor doing things for them! If you don't take care of yourself, then you are doing nobody a favor.

Please take care of yourself for the sake of you. Take care of yourself also for the sake of others. Make your health and well-being your utmost priority. Set the strongest boundaries around your own needs, and don't let anyone take your chance for pleasure away.

If you can squeeze another 10% out of your day, or even just five minutes, it is mandatory that you don't spend that precious time on your "To Do" list. Focus instead on your "To Be" list for balance.

To Be or To Do, That Is the Question

Everyone has a "To Do" list. Even if you don't actually sit down and record your daily chores, we know you have stuff to do. You need to get food, go to work and do the laundry. This is life.

We also know this: You need a "To Be" list too. In order to live a balanced life you will want to spend some of your hard earned time working toward being who you are meant to be. Nobody, ever, said at the end of their life that they wish they did one more load of laundry! We are willing to spend 95% of our time on our "To Do" list, but how many of us spend even a moment on our "To Be" list? How many of us ever spend a few moments a day contemplating if we are on the right track?

This much we know for sure: All that "To Do" stuff will still be there even if you take just a few minutes for yourself. We guarantee it! If you take five minutes to meditate, you will still have to pick up the kids. If you enjoy a cup of tea, you will still have to write that report. If you lay down for just 10 minutes, everything you need to do will still be waiting.

Isn't it comforting to know that some things don't change?
To bring balance to your life and to your day, create a "To Be" list. Make sure you are spending at least a little time and effort on being who you want to be. Write down the values you want to cultivate in your life. If you don't know where to begin, start with a generic list. Here are a few ideas:

Qualities to Cultivate on the Road to Balance and Joy

Adventure, *Altruism*, **Change**, *Commitment*, **Companionship**, Confidence Creativity, Discipline, **Education.** Emotional Security, FAITH, **Family,** FINANCIAL SECURITY, FORGIVENESS, *Freedom*, Friendship, **Fulfillment, Fun,** GROWTH, *Happiness,* **Health.** *Honesty.* Hope, **Humor,** Independence, INtegRity, *Kindness*, Knowledge, Love, **Peace of Mind,** *Progress.* **Reason, SECURITY,** *Self-Empowerment,* Self-Love, SELF-CARE, *Self-Reliance,* **Service,** Spirituality, Steadiness, **STRENGTH**, SUCCESS, **Truth,** Wisdom

---

We both do this work too. For nearly 20 years, Desiree has spent more than 150 days every year on the road, traveling all over the world teaching yoga. Part of her prescription for balance is that she mostly practices yoga alone when she is home. "Even an extreme extrovert like myself needs to recharge at times," she points out. "Practicing quietly is a ritual that I look forward to. And it makes me a better teacher when I am on the road." She is also a new wife, a new grandmother, and like many of us who are getting older, she is facing new challenges with her health and stamina.

Desiree's "To Be" List:

Strong, *Healthy,* **Content,** *Kind,* Patient, *Accepting,* *Available.* Responsive, Loving *and* *Positive*

Michelle, on the other hand, has a different set of needs. Her health was dramatically transformed in 2015. When she was ill, she was of no use to anybody, least of all to her family. She wants to stay healthy to serve the ones she loves and to participate fully in life.

Michelle's "To Be" List:

Healthy, Steady, *Strong,* **Trusting,** *Spiritual,* *Loving,* **Honest** *and* OPEN

Once you have your "To Be" list, then you will be able to prioritize your life. Remember, we are not talking about when to pick up the dry cleaning. We are talking about finding time to meet your own needs, being the person you want to be, and then everything else.

Desiree tells us, "Even when I'm on the road, I speak to my daughter and my husband at least by text every day. This fills up my 'loving' cup." And no matter where Desiree is in the world, she is almost always available to her family via technology. "For some people, they may see technology as an intrusion. But for me, it helps me feel connected. I need to feel close to my loved ones in order for me to provide support to people all around the world in my workshops. That's my balance."

On the other hand, Michelle works at home and has perfected the art of helicoptering around her family. She admits if she was more connected, they would stage an intervention. Therefore, she has a different priority: avoiding depression and taking care of her health. Some may see taking the time to exercise and build strength as a selfish endeavor, but for Michelle, it is the key to long-term joy. "I make my well-being a priority. I stop whatever I'm doing every day to make an hour or two to support my health—whether it's yoga, exercise, or walking the dog. If I can't possibly fit it in, I am very grouchy and nobody wants to be around me."

What People Want

When we talk about feeling out of balance, it's often related to either not having what we want, or not appreciating what we have. It's also the difference between how we spend our time, and how we'd like to spend our time. If so many people are unhappy because they don't have what they want, we were curious about what it is that most people want? Here is a list, in case you're curious too.

America's How-To Obsession

The top things Americans want,
according to the people who study such things:

1. *Flat Abs*
2. *Lose weight*
3. *Good skin*
4. *To age gracefully*
5. *Clean closets*
6. *Organized minds*
7. *Get rich*
8. *Better sleep*
9. *Happiness*
10. *Friends*

Consciousness Happens

The key to getting what you want and feeling more in balance is creating consciousness around your day and making yourself a priority. Habits don't just happen. We have to make them happen. Behavioral psychology tells us there are three "R's" to undertaking a new habit: Make a reminder to do it. Make it part of your routine. And create a reward for doing the behavior.

Ask yourself, what are you looking for? Can you think creatively about a solution to something you want to change? Can you take just a small step? Can you adjust your expectations from wanting ecstatic bliss to being okay? Can you establish a ritual? Are you able make it a habit? Can you support it with strong boundaries? Can you reward yourself for this new behavior?

Perfect. We've just solved the First World problem of finding balance in life. Onward.

The Inner Life

In yoga, there are two sides to a pose: how it feels and how it looks. On the outside, we may struggle to touch our toes for years, or to find the shape of a backbend that looks more like a perfect arc than a flattened pancake. But inside our poses can feel magnificent. They can be liberating and exhilarating, although to the common eye they may appear to be no big deal.

In this case, the eye misses the beauty of yoga. The richness and splendor of any pose happens on the inside, which is hard to see. It is how it makes us feel. The "perfect" pose is the one that may not look the best, yet it brings us that much closer to our "To Be" list. It can elicit a feeling of possibility and reward us for our perseverance.

It is the rare photo that can capture the essence of a pose and not just the shape. If we could see how it feels to the yogi, then we could understand the beauty of yoga. If we concentrate only on how a pose looks, then we miss half the practice of the inner life.

In this way, as we age, our inner life becomes much more important than what is happening on the outside. Perhaps when we are younger, we can pursue the poses like a circus competition. We go, go, go. Although in many cases as we age, we will start to become stiffer or less strong. If we could wake up and pop into a handstand at age 30, we may need coffee first when we're 60. In this way, the practice of yoga becomes much more beautiful to the older yogi. We now can learn to appreciate what cannot be seen when we had our youth and vitality. We take more notice of the steps on the path, and we're less focused on where it leads.

It Gets Better

Yoga, ultimately, is a path inward. Everything we seek about life: who we are, our dharma or our destiny resides inside. If the outside shape of the poses we practice on the mat is less than what we had anticipated, then the inside feeling of abundance is much more.

There is simply no explaining it until you feel it. How can a backbend pose, such as Wheel, that once may have resembled a mountain peak rising from the valley and now looks like a squatty hill, feel even better as we age? It gets better because of a vast amount of appreciation. The inner life of a pose is fueled by gratitude and resilience. At this point in our lives, we take nothing for granted in our yoga practice. At midlife and beyond, everything becomes a miracle! Everything we accomplish is a wonder.

Yoga teaches us to experience a pose, and therefore experience life from the inside out. We learn to work toward it, to be thankful for it, to understand it, and come to peace with it. It is very much like a long-term relationship we embark on with our body, mind, and spirit. If we only focus on the outside shape, then we miss the point of the practice.

Aging helps refocus us on the inner life. What the pose looks like on the outside is merely the act of coloring in the lines. By keeping our inner life rich and present, it is less likely we'll be completely knocked off balance when our hectic world sends us a curve ball. We know where to go to find that snippet of calm.

The Inner Life Is the Infinite Game

If life is a game, then we want to play as long as possible. Arnold Palmer, for example, played golf, designed courses and remained in the game throughout his entire life. We want to be the Arnold Palmers of living exceptionally well! We want to remain vibrant and vital long after dusk. The trick is learning how to *play* the game, and not just to *win*. "Golf is deceptively simple and endlessly complicated," Palmer said. The same is true of yoga and life.

If we play to *win* at the yoga pose, to do it the best, or to touch our feet to our heads, or some other measure of success, we are surely going to lose.

Three things will happen if you keep going after the pose, especially the hardest poses, relentlessly over time: You will hit a plateau. You will become injured. You will get older or your body will fail you.

We have a choice. Instead of playing to win where there is always a loser, we can play to grow better. In this way, we continue to win. "There are at least two kinds of games," wrote James Carse in his best-selling book, *The Finite and Infinite Game*. "A finite game is played for the purpose of winning, an infinite game for the purpose of continuing the play."

The purpose of yoga is about continuing the play. We want to balance out life's ups and downs by simply showing up. We look to make *progress*, not to be perfect. If we only wanted to "do" a yoga pose, then most likely we would give up. But if we look to *feel* it, to be hopeful on the inside, to find the gratitude in the moment, then we keep going.

There is simply no getting around a certain loss of strength and flexibility as we age. If we cling to the outcome of a pose, we are probably going to lose. Most certainly we'll miss out on the internal feeling of a posture. If we can set our sights on a broader view of staying in the game, then we can be like Diana Nyad, the Olympic swimmer. We will have a body that's almost as strong, with a much more resilient mind. #Winning!

Stepping Back and Out with Meditation

According to the *Yoga Sutras*, the intent of yoga is to quiet the mind. Everything we do, the postures, the practice, the purpose, is simply to experience a peaceful mind, free of the turmoil of life.

It is not easy, but it is attainable.

If the outer world is chaotic, it will usually set your mind to racing. However, if you can calm the mind, then you are better equipped to deal with the pandemonium and unpredictability of life. If our mind and spirit are also a confused, muddled mess, then there is no chance to attain equanimity.

Yoga Chitta Vritti Nirodha

Yoga is the cessation of the fluctuations of the mind.
~ **Yoga Sutras of Patanjali, 1.2**

Benefits of Meditation

There are close to 80 well-documented physical, psychological and emotional benefits of meditation. But most importantly, sitting quietly for just five minutes can allow you to stop whatever you are doing. Stop and drop in! We are a society of go, go, go, so a hard stop is what we need to bring balance. Meditate to rejuvenate.

These are just a few documented benefits of meditation:

Sit quietly to ...

- *Reduce stress*
- *Improve focus and concentration*
- *Develop self-awareness and self-acceptance*
- *Increase a sense of happiness*
- *Slow all of the effects of aging*
- *Benefit cardiovascular and immune health*
- *Counteract ADHD symptoms*
- *Be a better parent, friend, lover, and human being*

It's true. Meditation can do all these things and more. When Desiree and Michelle had small children, they thought time outs were for parents! "Whenever I took a couple of deep breaths and paused, everything calmed down," Michelle said. "I don't know if I was a better parent, but nobody got hurt."

Desiree has, by her own admission, never been a good meditator. "Sitting on a pillow with my eyes closed only gave my already very quick mind license to race around like a crazed stallion. My mind is like Netflix™ on Speed, constantly bringing me old movies to watch."

So in 2016 she decided to attend a 10-day silent Vipassana retreat. This opportunity and gift to herself provided Desiree with new coping skills to help with several issues, including her lasting sorrow over losing her son. It is not easy to schedule the time away from one's normal life. Yet she felt it was worth it to find peace of mind.

"I now have another way to deal with my loss and pain," she explains. "Meditation is a tool. It helped me realize that I want to spend less time in misery, less time spinning the stories of blame and shame. I needed to learn how to do this for myself, so that I can help others who have experienced similar heartbreak. In many ways, I feel this is to be my life's work."

If you are starting a meditation practice, whatever you can do will produce results. Even if you can be quiet for just two minutes, then you are two minutes better off than before. If you can't sit unsupported yet, then lie down for a *Savasana*, or quiet nap-like meditation. If you can only close your eyes for five breaths, then you are five breaths closer to calm. When it comes to meditation, the ritual is more important than the result. And no effort, not even a second, is wasted.

Physical Balance Is Also Critical

After we pursue the balance of a healthy inner life, a peaceful mind, experiencing joy, and an abundant sense of gratitude for what is, we want to remember that the purely physical sense of balance also begins to deteriorate as we age.

Blame it on our brains. According to the National Institutes of Health, 33 million adults in America seek medical care every year for balance-related issues including dizziness, nausea, ringing in the ears (tinnitus), and vertigo. There are specific scientific and medical causes for why we lose our balance more as we age. Our inner ear structure starts to deteriorate, as well as the part of our brain that controls our sense of space. At some point in our lives, we could have been exposed to a virus. Our necks also grow weaker, which also affects the inner ear and the cervical spine, putting our delicate nervous system at risk.

However, we also lose our balance because we don't use it. As children at a playground or at school we used to stand on one leg, play hopscotch, hang from a monkey bar by one arm, jump rope, and so on. But as adults, we rarely practice balancing for more than the second it takes to put one foot in front of the other or put on our pants. That's how it is. But we can do better than that.

Balance is a use it or lose it situation. It is just like any physical skill or speaking a foreign language. You must use it or your brain simply forgets how.

So even if you say, "I have no balance," you must absolutely practice balancing. Hold a chair or a wall until you can maintain balance on your own. It will come back. Start with one to three seconds, working up to 30-second holds. Stand on one leg, rise up on your toes, lean way forward and lean way back. Try the yoga Tree Pose; then try it with a backbend. Any place you begin is a good place to start.

"My balance today is much better than it was when I was younger," said Marc, a 50-year-old yogi from Denver. "I was terribly uncoordinated as a child, but since I've been practicing yoga for 15 years now, my balance is actually very good."

The Practice:
Balance is Loving All of It

Wrists and Hands

If we are balanced we are able to use all of our body to support our weight. This includes our core and even our hands. We cannot hang in our postures and dump weight into the wrists. As we age, our wrists can weaken and repetitive motions can also take its toll. We need to use the "all of it" to find balance along the way.

Strengthening

- Spend time squeezing a hard or semi-hard ball that fits into your palm.

- Tabletop on a Block. On all fours, place your hands flat on two blocks in front of you. Bring your wrists off the block but keep your knuckles on top. Try to lift and lower the arms, without using the thumbs, just your forearm muscles. Graduate to doing this in Downward Facing Dog.

- Down Dog. Practice pressing your finger pads down more firmly and lifting your arms up rather than dumping weight into your wrists.

- "Finger" Balances. All arm balances and inversions require strong hands. Test your strength by coming to your fingertips. A little goes a long way.

Stretching

- Shake and massage your hands. A lot.

- Stretch your fingers. One at a time, pull them out and stretch them forward and back.

- Stretch your wrists. Hold one of your hands with the other and pull down as far as you can go, both forward and back, keeping your fingers straight.

- Tabletop Stretch. On all fours, turn your hands around so your fingers are facing back toward you and gently stretch your wrists. Move slightly forward and back.

Yoga Poses for Wrists

Strengthen your hands and wrists to maintain dexterity and balance.

Downward Facing Dog, *Adho Mukha Svanasana*
Downward Facing Dog is often a main cause of wrist pain. Practice lifting up and out of your core, rather than dumping weight into the back of the wrists.

Yoga Push Up, *Chaturanga*
Chaturanga also strengthens the wrists. Try the entire
sequence from Downward Dog, to High Plank, to
Chaturanga, to Low Plank, to Upward Facing Dog
solely on the ridges of the hands.

Wheel, *Urdvha Dhanurasana*
Wheel is a challenging pose. Desiree has been known to do
up to 108 at a time. Michelle is overjoyed to do three in a
week. It's a test of strength, perseverance, open shoulders,
open quads and flexible wrists. Begin by lying on the floor
with your feet near your hips. Place your hands by your
head, fingers toward your heels. Lift your torso, hips and
head off the floor. Be sure to keep your arms parallel and
your shoulders on your back. If this is too much on the
wrists, then place your hands on tilted blocks near a wall.
That will relieve the pressure until you have developed
more strength and flexibility.

Gorilla, *Uttanasana Variation*
In Standing Forward Fold, place both hands underneath
your feet, palms upward. Then press gently. Turn the hands
around and do the other side.

Peacock, *Mayurasana*
Peacock Pose is the ultimate wrist strengthener and arm
balance. From Tabletop on all fours, place your hands on
the mat. Then turn them around so the fingers face backward. Squeeze the elbows together and slowly place your
ribs on top of them. Lean forward placing more weight on
your forearms until your legs come off the ground.

Grace	Pose	Grit
Play with lifting the wrists	Handstand	On the ridgetops or fingertips, at a wall
Kneeling, lean forward	Peacock	Head and legs off the ground
Place hands on blocks at a wall	Wheel	Press arms and/or legs straight

Life is a balance between grace and grit.
To see a video tutorial of these poses, go to
www.YogaDownload.com

Fearless After Fifty: Practical Advice Too busy? Not for this!

Easy and inexpensive
These tiny changes will make a big difference in your life.

- Start every day with 16 oz. of warm water with the juice of one lemon.

- Stretch your spine six ways, shoulders and hips in all directions.

- Walk to lunch, to the grocery, down the hall.

- Massage your feet and sensitive joints.

- Stand at your desk rather than sit.

- Balance on one leg while you are waiting to check out at the grocery store.

- Do squats while you are reading labels at the store.

- Lift hand weights while using the speakerphone.

More ... money, time and focus

- Test for food sensitivities. You might feel terrible and the answer is as simple as cutting out certain foods. Dairy, Soy, Wheat, Gluten, Sugar, Nightshade Vegetables, and Alcohol have all been proven, no question about it, to be inflammatory.

- Wear a step monitor and consciously increase your movement.

- Track your food intake with one of the many mobile apps.

- See a nutritionist and fine-tune your diet.

- Focus on sleep. Create a ritual. If you stay up late, then plan a way to make up for the deficit. Sleep is an essential requirement to function at your peak.

- Take a meditation class or download a variety of guided meditations.

- Try Tai Chi or another mind/body moving meditation.

- Commit to a yoga practice on a daily or weekly basis.

All in!

- Book an exercise vacation at a luxury spa.

- Sign up for a meditation retreat.

- Book a silent retreat.

- To jump-start a healthy eating habit, visit a health center such as Pritikin or the Mayo Clinic.

- Attend a meditation seminar.

Eight
Plan B

*The most successful people
are those who are good at Plan B.*
~ James A. Yorke

Plan B is what the Universe has in mind.

Desiree set out to be a dancer. She had her heart set on modern dance, performing across America and opening a studio. Well, today she is an international yoga teacher.

Michelle loved to ski and ride horses. Her family moved to Colorado so they could ski 30 days a year. And then her knees became a problem. Of course, if it's not one thing, it's two others. So then she broke her neck.

We know what it is to love something madly, and then either not be any good at it, or not be able to do it anymore. Things change, especially as we age, but it could be for the better.

Being fearless, steady and strong *all through our lives* is about finding new loves and new passions when life throws us a curve ball. Knowing that change happens, we acknowledge that our body, mind and spirit will transform over time. So how can we learn to find the same thrill in what we can do, and not seek it in what we can't?

"Loving what you have is truly the secret to happiness," Desiree explains.

Happy Accidents

It was chance that brought Michelle to yoga. She started riding competitively when she was just four years old. Yet 40 years later her back hurt so much that she had to give it up. A physical therapist suggested Pilates, but on her way to the class she got lost and ended up in yoga.

"When I started yoga, it was to build my strength so I could get back to riding," Michelle points out. "But I began to feel the same passion and commitment to yoga as I did to horses. I just didn't have the time to spend at a barn anymore. Yoga was a much more manageable way to find passion in life."

Happy ending? Not so much. Michelle still loved horses! She always thought as soon as her kids went to college she would ride again. But then the Universe intervened and she fractured two vertebrae in her neck. This meant that if she were to fall, the fragile bones might fully break.

"I had to figure this out. Being miserable is not an option!" Then one day in 2016 she received an email from a local horse rescue center. They needed volunteers to help with newly acquired horses, many of which were starving and sick. It was a godsend. "Now I use my passion and equestrian skills to nurture these animals. I've never been so happy in a barn in all my life."

Thank you, Universe

The same was true for Desiree. Lucky for us, she found her way to yoga, but it wasn't her first choice for a career.

"My first love was modern dance," she said. "Yet after years of practice and performance, my body was beginning to break down. I turned to yoga to heal my body, but the surprising thing was it also nurtured my spirit."

There is always a chance that Desiree would have become a world famous dancer, performing in companies in New York or San Francisco. Even if that had happened, how long could it have lasted? We'll never know. Instead, her talents were diverted to yoga. Now she travels the world teaching and changing the lives of thousands of people and has no plans to quit in midlife. Indeed, there are not many dancers still *en pointe* at 50!

Plan B is funny that way.

The Universe's Option

When plans don't turn out the way we hoped, it could be for the best. These moments are often the turning points in our lives and should not be missed. Instead of wasting time yearning for what was, we could choose to pay attention to what is, because we guarantee that at some point, things will not go our way. How can we best use our talents, skills and passion to find happiness, to serve, to transform the lives of others and positively change the world?

Many events shape our lives forever altering who we are. When things go off the rails, it's hard to see it as a gift. When we see our loved ones suffer, or perhaps we lose a job, or we have to redefine our purpose, we experience these moments as the most trying and mystifying of times. Yet it could turn out better.

The Universe could be conspiring for you ....

Aging Changes Everything

There is nothing quite like the aging process. It is inexplicable to someone who isn't going through it. We are literally not ourselves anymore. Our bodies change and so do our capacities. At times it feels like body, mind, and spirit have been abducted by aliens! There might also come a time when doing what we love actually becomes unloving to ourselves. Then what?

Yoga.

Yoga teaches us to pay attention. By being focused on the mat, it helps us see clearly in other areas of our lives. It teaches us perseverance. Understand, you are not meant to be "good at yoga." You are never meant to "master" a pose, because the poses can always be made harder or deeper, and your body continually changes. Yoga teaches us patience and compassion. One day you have a pose, and the next day, poof, it's gone. Yoga teaches us that we're not in charge, and that's okay. Then you try again, and little by little you start to see results in your effort. This gives you hope and a little swagger in your step.

Aging wakes us up. The fluctuations in our body, mind, and spirit let us know that things are not the same. Aging creates an awareness, as well as a sense of urgency in our purpose. After all, time is running out.

It might be time to ask ourselves the important questions. What are we meant to do? What is our intention? And most importantly, how can we serve? We want to stay relevant in the world. At this point, you may need to upgrade not just your electronics, but also your view of how you fit into the great scheme of things.

Start by asking yourself, "What matters to me?" It's that simple. Usually we dwell on, "What's the matter with me?" But it's much more important to figure out what matters to you, and then find a way to contribute.

A Fish Story

The greatest fish story of all time was about a whale named *Moby Dick*. Captain Ahab was obsessed with the great white whale. Nothing else would do; he had to have this whale. Spoiler alert: like many obsessions, this one ends badly.

In real life we also pursue our fish. We have our passions and our nemesis, and we don't seem to know when to let go.

Michelle saw this in her late father-in-law, who was an avid fisherman all his life. He grew up fishing in northern Canada, Minnesota, and Montana and loved Walleye Pike. In 2005, he moved to Colorado to be close to his grandchildren. Little did any of us know that warmer temperatures during the past 50 years meant that Walleye either no longer existed or were very hard to find in the more southern regions.

"He spent months bemoaning that the rivers and streams in Colorado did not have Walleye," Michelle points out. "Colorado happens to be home to a huge sport fishing industry for Cutthroat, Rainbow, Brown, Brook and Lake trout, Kokanee Salmon and Mountain Whitefish. But not Walleye."

From the outside, we can see that perhaps her father-in-law might have enjoyed fishing for something else, if it was the activity that he loved. But instead, he focused on how much he missed this fish.

In yoga, we call this separating the fruits of our actions from the action itself. We learn that joy is contained in the practice. We take pleasure in showing up. Persistence is the key. The pleasure is not actually the pose; it's in the activity itself. To find joy, to cultivate happiness, we only need to fish, to practice, and to do it over and over again simply for the delight of it.

Sri Patabhi Jois reminds us, "Practice, and all is coming." The secret to life, to being happy, to finding satisfaction and joy is simply to fish, not necessarily to catch the fish.

Many men go fishing all of their lives
without knowing that it is not fish they are after.
~ Henry David Thoreau

What We Know for Sure

Experienced yogis know this to be true. If you work all your life to get a pose, you might get it. Or you might not. Or you might get it just once, and then it's gone again.

"There are yoga fairies," explains David Swenson, the Ashtanga teacher, "that know exactly which pose you really want, so they let you have it. Once. And then they take it away."

If we're not careful, "the pose" can become our great white whale, our Moby Dick or Walleye Pike. We can go after it all we want, but we'll never have the same satisfaction as the person who knows it's not the pose they are after.

The real teaching of yoga and the practice is this: We practice for the sake of practice. We do this thing not to get a fish, but to get a life.

Finding Joy

Sometimes it's hard to figure out what really matters to us. We can become fixated on the wrong things. To get to the heart of this dilemma, write down an answer to these questions:

What Matters to You?

- *What makes you happy?*
- *What would you do, if you could do anything?*
- *How do you spend your free time?*
- *How does that make you feel?*
- *When do you feel exhilarated?*

Now look at what you've written. If it's not a "fish" that you are looking for, then what is it?

"I wish I knew to do this simple work way back when I couldn't ride horses anymore," explains Michelle. "I spent much too much time mourning the loss of something I loved, which stood in the way of being happy with what I had."

"Volunteering at the horse barn has been the most amazing experience," she admits. "I feel much more useful loving and caring for these animals than I ever did riding. One action takes pleasure for myself, and the other gives it. There is no comparison in how it makes you feel. It is the best of all possibilities. I am useful, and most of all, my knees don't ache when I'm done."

It was a change in her body that brought Desiree to yoga as well. It was a case of teacher, heal thyself. "I found my way to yoga in my late 20s at a time when my dance performances and my yoga practice overlapped," Desiree tells us. "Though

I loved the exhilaration of the dance, I quickly came to see that performing was taking a tremendous toll on my body, and that yoga was always healing or fixing my aches, sprains, and minor stress fractures. At the time I was also teaching dance and as I looked to the future, I could see that even though these dancers enjoyed what they were doing, I would be able to offer more to my students if I taught them how to use yoga to heal themselves."

Desire continues to be inspired by the healing power of yoga for a person's body and mind, and sharing it has been her passion. "For me, there is no better feeling than being able to offer what I have learned and experienced in order to help someone else."

Arthritis Is a Game Changer

If you are in midlife or even approaching your 40s, if nothing else has slowed you down, eventually that constraint could be arthritis. It was pain in her joints that interrupted Desiree's dance career. It was arthritis that ultimately caused Michelle to break multiple bones in her body.

There are 350 million people worldwide, and 50 million in the United States who suffer from doctor-diagnosed arthritis and inflammation disease, according to the Arthritis Foundation. Economically, that accounts for $156 billion annually in lost wages and medical expenses and nearly one million hospitalizations. But what does it do to the spirit of a once-active person? You guessed it. Arthritis can be devastating.

We are the active generation! We expect to remain strong and vibrant throughout our entire lives. We grew up running and jumping and testing our mettle. We are the age that came of age with Title Nine and women's professional sports. And that's exactly how arthritis became so pervasive and we got into this mess.

What slowing down teaches us is that when the body fails, the spirit can still soar.

Yoga Thrills

When Michelle could no longer take a horse over a fence, and when Desiree could no longer dance without pain, they each had to discover another way to have that thrill in the veins. "I wasn't ready to give up," said Desiree.

At first, both of them had to heal. The beauty of yoga is that it can meet you where you are. If you need to heal your back, or become stronger in your legs, it can provide the tools that will assist you in doing that. If you need to relieve pain, yoga can do that too.

Yoga can also be your Plan B. If you're looking for adventure, practice inversions. If you are looking for steadiness, practice long holds. If you are looking for balance, practice postures that build stability.

Believe us when we say, whatever you want, whatever you need, you can find it on the mat.

Fearless After Fifty: The Practice: Stepping Back with Meditation

Meditation and Restorative Poses

You would think that sitting would be easy, but sitting properly requires a strong back, a connected core, and a lifted seat to maintain lumbar support. If a pose isn't comfortable, it won't be restorative.

Strengthening

The Pelvis and *Mula Bandha*

Strengthen the pelvic floor with *Mula Bandha* (pelvic lock). Contract the pelvic floor upward from the perineum. In women, it is similar to a Kegel-type exercise.

The Abdominals and *Uddiyana Bandha*

Strengthen the core with *Uddiyana Bandha* (abdominal lock). Lean slightly forward and suck your stomach up and in. Hold for a few seconds before letting out the air.

The Head and Neck, *Jalandhara Bandha* (chin lock)

Even if you are resting in restorative poses, it is important that you maintain proper alignment. You do not want your head lolling forward, placing undue stress on the spine. *Jalandhara Bandha* will strengthen the neck. Contract the throat muscles and tilt the head forward so that the chin touches the chest very high, between the two collarbones. Hold the breath and the pose for a few seconds before relaxing and letting out the air.

Stretching for Meditation

Spinal Stretch

Prepare the spine for a seated meditation by stretching it in all four directions. In "Easy Seat," or cross-legged, place one hand in front and one in back. Twist in both directions, maintaining a tall spine and a lumbar curve. Then sit on one hand, reach the opposite hand up and over the head, stretching the side of the spine. Repeat on the other side.

Meditation

When preparing for a seated meditation, alignment is crucial. You cannot relax or restore if you are in pain. If there is discomfort, use support or lie down. That you find a moment of peace and quiet far outweighs how you get there.

Sit cross-legged. Always use a cushion or blanket when sitting on the floor for an anterior tilt of the pelvis and to maintain the natural lumbar curve. If your knees are much higher than the pelvis, then sit on an even bigger "throne." In this case, comfort is king.

Use your core to maintain steady support, yet do not overly engage the muscles. Keep an awareness of your head to maintain an upright position, not drifting forward or back.

Yoga Poses for Meditation

Supported Hero's Pose, *Virasana*

If sitting in "Easy Seat" is not comfortable, then try supported *Virasana*. Sit on top of a bolster or blocks, kneeling, with the soles of your feet behind you, facing up. Use a blanket to keep the lumbar curve so the spine, including your neck, will naturally be more balanced and upright.

In meditation practice, notice your breath, deepening both the inhalations and exhalations. Make use of music or chanting, candles or incense to inspire your quiet time. Watch your thoughts and notice that you have the power to dwell on them or not. Eventually you will be able to move from your day-to-day thoughts to a broader sense of connectedness with the Universe.

Legs Up the Wall, *Viparita Karani*

Viparita Karani is our favorite restorative pose, hands down, or legs up! Place a yoga mat perpendicular to a wall. Maneuver your body to get as close to the wall as possible, then flip onto your back and bring your legs up the wall. For extra lumbar support and to create a small curve, you can place a blanket under your sacrum. Let your arms rest with bent elbows, like a cactus plant, to lift your heart. Your blood and lymph glands will drain out of your feet and legs and move toward your heart and lungs where it will be cleaned. Come out of the pose slowly. You will feel refreshed both mentally and physically.

Child's Pose, *Balasana*
Sitting on your heels, widen the knees and fold forward placing your hands on the ground. Child's Pose can restore your sense of composure and ease. Try rounding forward onto a bolster for extra support.

There is no sliding scale from Grace to Grit, because these poses are all Grace.

Before we can love others, we must first love ourselves.
To see a video tutorial of these poses,
go to *www.YogaDownload.com*

Fearless After Fifty: Practical Advice How to Stay Relevant

Easy and inexpensive
Volunteer! Nothing feels like purpose more than serving.
- Ask yourself, what matters to you?

More ... money, time and focus
- Embrace technology. Take a computer course.
- Learn about Facebook, Pinterest, Twitter, and other social media sites.

- Be flexible. The Universe may bring you something you hadn't considered before.

- Reach out. Contact your former work associates and see if there's a way to get involved.

- Listen! Sometimes people talk more and listen less. Don't be that person.

All in!

- Start a Foundation.

- Serve on a Board of Directors.

- Go back to work.

- Keep learning. To stay relevant you must stay interested. Go back to school, take a course, read, write, mentor.

- Teach yourself a new skill.

- Invest in a new look. Nothing says "out of date" like having the same hairstyle, clothes, and shoes for 40 years. Change up the outside, and the inside will change too.

Nine
Our Time to Thrive

We must make the most of every living moment.
~ Jackie Kennedy Onassis

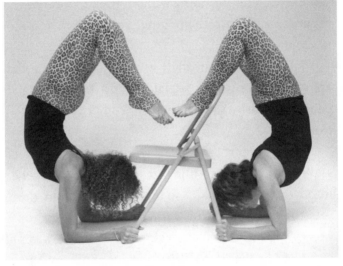

Scorpion

Midlife means we are halfway, on the way home. This is the time to choose our game plan for the second half. Do we want the "normal" human experience, where we reach our peak in our forties and then experience a slow decline until the end? Or do we want something more?

We believe we all want to flourish, feel useful, have purpose to our lives, and grow better, wiser and stronger every day. In a nutshell, we wish to thrive. To do this, it takes commitment and courage. We do not want to let our fears about what's to come stop us from living fully in the now. For support, we want to find like-minded people. We do not do well in isolation. In fact, isolation is a common method of torture.

For instance, Sebastian Junger documented the effects on soldiers and others when they returned from war in his book, *Tribe*. He found that while combat was grim, often the real trauma was coming home without the support of a tight-knit group or a sense of belonging. Feeling lost and alone was worse than war.

"Humans are so strongly wired to help one another—and enjoy such enormous social benefits from doing so—that people regularly risk their lives for complete strangers," Junger explains.

From the start, *Fearless After Fifty* has been an act of labor and love primarily to find our tribe. When Michelle walked into Desiree's workshop so many years ago, she thought she was the only one who wanted to "find more" out of life. Meeting Desiree was the validation that she was no longer alone. Michelle tells us, "The day I saw another woman my age going for it, saying, 'You can do this,' and actually believing in me, was incredible. I almost cried. In fact, I think I did."

"We are expected to reach our highpoint somewhere in early adulthood, then slowly decline into our 80s," Desiree confirms. "Well, I never wanted the normal human experience. I want to thrive every single day, well into my 80s and beyond."

We want to squeeze every bit of pleasure out of every moment, for all of the days of our lives. Yoga helps us to be present, to be awake and aware, to be healthy and happy, and it paves the way for better health in our later years.

And yet, we have been raised to think that midlife means the beginning of the end of life. We have news for you: It's not game over. It's game on. "It's easier to believe the fear around aging and that going downhill is the natural route," Desiree said. "It is an excuse to let go and give up, when the going gets tough."

Michelle adds, "It's easier to tell an older yogi, 'Be careful, Grandma. You don't want to hurt yourself.' It takes time and patience to work with older students, to help them find their potential, and to build and strengthen muscles. If you work strong, you get strong."

If you attempt a handstand or an arm balance, and you can't do it, we like to think, "Oh, you can't do that yet," or "You haven't been practicing that long enough." There is always another day to get on your mat and try.

"The truth is, everyone, at every stage, at every age, in every circumstance can start to live a better life and find more of what they're looking for in yoga," Desiree acknowledges. "You have to start with attitude, and the rest naturally follows. Laughing at yourself and turning a deaf ear to the naysayers helps, too!"

Aging well is mostly an experience of the spirit, since the body is going to do what the body is going to do. We can't stop what happens on a cellular level or change what we see in a mirror. Abundance and expansion begin inside, with our resilient spirit, and then that is supported by community.

Since Desiree started the Wisdom Warriors yoga training in 2012 she has met hundreds of other like-minded midlife beings who still want to be strong and vital. Men and women tell her, "I thought I was the only one." You are not alone. There are others out there who are craving a sense of belonging, perhaps while standing on their hands. It would be lonely and discouraging to try and stay strong and vital while the whole world chimes in that to even have such a dream is ridiculous.

As Junger described, we have your back. We have shared goals and shared dreams. We don't want the normal human experience! We want something more.

Desiree's Vision

Aging is possibly the hardest challenge we will ever have to find abundance on a path that feels more limited and difficult by the day. It's not our imaginations that our capabilities begin to falter, our mental acuity starts to waver, and even our muscle mass shrinks. So we absolutely need to know that we are supported in this process.

"My dream is to build a place where I am surrounded by a like-minded community," explains Desiree. "I want to live near my kind of people."

Today Desiree travels around the world, many times over, to see her dearest friends and yoga community. She's been to every continent and even taught in Abu Dhabi where under the *burkha*, we women are the same beings.

Wherever she teaches, she's met by people who say, "You give me hope."

"It is truly life-affirming," said Desiree. But these days she is feeling the pull of family, a new granddaughter, and the desire to stay home more often.

"I love finding 'my people' all over the world. But my dream is a place where we all live close enough to practice together on the mat, and seek out the best in health and wellness not just for a vacation, but as a lifestyle."

During the past few years Desiree and her husband, Andrew Rivin, have hosted a two-week summer camp for adults in Southern California. Her dream is to expand this to the other 50 weeks of the year!

"Everyone needs like-minded beings around to thrive," she declares. "I would love to have mine around me more often."

Take Care of Your Temple

A more traditional or Vedantic Hindu approach to yoga maintains that the body is ignoble and undeserving of love, and that only the spirit is worthy. We take a more modern, Tantric view. We see the body as our temple, and worthy of love and care because it keeps our spirit warm. Pain, illness and injury will bring a body down, and then the spirit, faster than you can say Jiminy Cricket.

To feel abundance, we want to make the physical body as healthy as possible. Instead of the body being unworthy, it is our sanctuary. It is our duty to keep our physical form in good health so our spirit may soar.

The Truth About Midlife

We want to sum up our attitude with 12 *Fearless After Fifty Midlife Realities*. You may not like all of them. Some of our "realities" may not be real or true for you at all. Some may be annoying or make you angry. Some may make you sad. Some you might be able use, and some you will discard. But we want to offer you what has worked for many who continue to grow better, stronger and more resilient every year.

FAF Midlife Reality #1: Start Now

The first most powerful words of the Yoga Sutras say this best:

Atha yoga anushasanam.
Now yoga begins.
~ **Yoga Sutra 1.1**

This is the most simple of truths: Now yoga begins. Not later. Not after we pick up the kids or drop off the dry cleaning. Not after that piece of cake. Not January 1. Now. You will never be younger, or better prepared, than you are at this moment. Embrace it.

We ask you to commit to changing your lifestyle, to be more active today than yesterday, so that all your tomorrows are better. Whenever you begin, you can immediately change the course of aging. Immediately.

When we are younger we can get by with less sleep and a poor diet, with nonstop days and extreme stress in our lives. In time, these kinds of choices will take their toll. Perhaps the lesson of having our body begin to wane is that we must now take more care with ourselves. We must now practice yoga.

FAF Midlife Reality #2:
Being Mindful Is Hard

Living a mindful life is difficult. It is easier to rush around being busy, busy, busy than to actually be present, awake and aware. Sometimes being conscious means being uncomfortable. It means being aware of the good and the bad. It means recognizing when we have done wrong and apologizing. It means forgiving and being forgiven. Ouch.

Be brave. Be present. Try not to dwell on the past and drive yourself crazy with things you cannot change. Try not to skip ahead to the future where you have to do a million things. Be willing to be present and let discomfort be the teacher. Being fully here in the moment is the only way to squeeze every bit of pleasure out of it. It's the only way to stop being afraid of the future. It's the only way to live a fearless life.

FAF Midlife Reality #3:
Making Ourselves a Priority Is Essential

Midlife often means that we have spent the first half of our lives ignoring our own needs in order to take care of everyone and everything else. We have been taught that to think of the self is selfish. We should be humble and serve. These are all useful values, of course! But now it's time for balance.

It's hard to hold those principles as absolute *and* take care of ourselves at the same time. That's how many of us got into this pickle of feeling "less than" as we age. We are exhausted! If we are going to have a better second half, then we need to find the balance between loving others and loving ourselves. Starting right now, create positive habits and rituals. Make time for what you are passionate about. Set boundaries. Teach others how you want to be treated; then hold them to it.

FAF Midlife Reality #4: Only You Can Do This

Nobody else can do the hard work of making your life better other than you. Begin each day with focus and intention.

Just like our computers and tablets, we need to start each day with a check of our operating system. Do a body scan, a spirit scan, a mind scan. Then assess what you need to bring yourself to a state of happiness.

We love the idea of a "body scan." Begin every morning with a new habit of giving yourself a once-over. How do you feel? What do you need? Sit quietly, take 10 conscious minutes in bed, go for a walk, or meditate to check in. It's much easier to get up and get going rather than being mindful. Even choosing perhaps to do cardio exercise on Monday and then yoga on Tuesday is an unconscious habit. See how you feel, then give yourself what you need. You do not have to be a victim of your life. Empower yourself to choose your path from this point on.

FAF Midlife Reality #5: The Going Will Get Tough

Humans are hardwired to avoid hard work. We invented the wheel to make life easier! We are programmed by nature to avoid the difficult stuff supported by our clever minds. Don't be a weenie! Be a winner. "Always be the hardest worker in the room," said Dwayne Johnson, aka the Rock.

Dive into your life. You don't need to pick and choose your experiences; be courageous and have the all of it. Take the good with the bad. Be willing to slow down and heal, then work hard again. Practice your yoga strong using every single muscle you got. Let life be one long wonder-ride of amazement so that at the end you know you gave it your all, and you didn't miss a thing.

FAF Midlife Reality #6: Choice Is Not Easy

We may say "choose happy," but we know choosing is not easy. It's our destiny to sometimes make poor decisions. So don't sweat it! You will make some good decisions, and you will make some that need revisiting sooner than you thought. What's more, for those of us who suffer from depression, it feels nearly impossible to choose "happy" at certain times.

Be willing to try. Start with a new habit of "yes," or at least "maybe." Find support. Reward yourself for positive behaviors. Embrace change as a way of choosing you.

FAF Midlife Reality #7: You Have To Believe

Faith is the first step, and yet so often it's the hardest one to take. You have to believe that you can be fearless. You have to trust that life gets better. The mind is a very unwilling believer. It is our "meddle-in-law." You must find a way to tell it to quiet down. You must find a way to let go of control and embrace what is. You have to believe that the Universe is conspiring for you. You ... Absolutely ... Must!

FAF Midlife Reality #8:
It's Body First, Then Mind and Spirit

The body is our temple and so it is our sacred duty to keep it healthy. It is very difficult to be comfortable and content if you abuse your body with alcohol, drugs and food. Taking care of our physical form also includes managing our weight. Of all the "realities," this is often the hardest.

Weight is one of the most sensitive issues to discuss in today's world, and yet at this moment, more than two-thirds of adults are overweight or medically obese, according to the National Institute for Diabetes. In other words, more of us cannot be at ease in the body than those who can.

As yoga teachers we don't want to say what is or is not a healthy weight for you. We feel that it is much more important to be happy with how you look and feel than it is to be at a number on a scale. A healthy weight is one that supports your lifestyle. That said, there are accepted medical definitions of what is a healthy weight. Your doctor probably has a table of acceptable heights and weights and recommendations as well.

But please, let's not kid ourselves. Being overweight is one of the primary factors for a multitude of illnesses including heart disease, arthritis, diabetes and cancer. It is also harder on our joints, ligaments and tendons. Love your body, but for the love of life, be healthy too.

Which brings us to food. You cannot thrive in any sense of the meaning if your body does not have the nutrition it needs to function at maximum capacity. While we are not nutritionists, we have strong feelings about what supports our bodily sanctuary.

"Food is a primary focus of my day," Desiree said. "It is my fuel, so I want to give myself the best energy producing substances I can. I love to spend time selecting, preparing, and then enjoying delicious, nutritious food."

Michelle also participated in a cleanse that changed how she viewed her diet and primary food sources. "I ate what I thought was clean, healthy food," she said. "However, after spending 21 days without gluten, sugar, dairy, eggs, caffeine, or alcohol, I have an entirely new understanding of what a whole food is, along with what nutrition can do for your body."

We don't want to tell you what to eat. We just want you to be more mindful. As aware as you become about your health and vigor, apply that consciousness and curiosity to the food you eat as well. As we age we start to lose muscle mass, so we may need to increase our consumption of protein. Sugar depletes energy. Pay attention to carbohydrates. Get an adequate supply of fiber and nutrients. Drink plenty of water. Try to eat something fresh at every meal, a piece of fruit or a vegetable. Avoid processed foods. Nutrients have been taken right out of the finished product, which leaves empty calories that do not fuel the body.

One trick to help you begin is to stay on the perimeter of the grocery store. The outside edge usually has the fresh meats, fish, vegetables, eggs and dairy. Processed foods are most often found in the center aisles.

FAF Midlife Reality #9: Take Baby Steps

Typically, we read a book about how to live fearlessly and we expect big results right away. We think we can practice one

Down Dog and we're fearless, badass midlife warriors. We wish it were that simple! It actually takes a million baby steps to get where we're going. First off, separate the results of your actions from the action itself, or in simple English, just do it, over and over again, for the love of it.

Start your day with the simplest step possible: Do a scan of your body, mind, and spirit. Then make a plan to incorporate the smallest change that will bring you closer to what you need. You wouldn't embark on a journey without a map, so why would you start your day without a plan? In time you may see transformation. The *Bhagavad Gita* tells us, "No effort is ever wasted." Not even a tiny one.

FAF Midlife Reality #10: It Takes Commitment and Discipline

Midlife means everything will get a tad harder to maintain: strength, flexibility and endurance. But we have a much better mind! We are seasoned now. We know about resilience and not giving up. We may be a beginner at yoga, but we can have a mature mind in how we approach something new.

One sure path to making a plan and sticking to it is to write it down. We are believers in journaling, although we know that writing down your feelings, wants and needs is not for everyone. Seeing your thoughts and desires on paper may be troublesome and perhaps inconvenient. It puts into words your deepest and most personal issues. Yet writing has also been shown to be healing, beneficial and redemptive. "Over the past few decades, the therapeutic power of writing has been discovered," Adrian Furnham, PhD, explains.[21] "People are encouraged first to learn to write, but then to tell their story."

After so many years tapping out notes on a computer, it may not even feel natural to start each day writing things the old-fashioned way. But the simple act of putting pen to paper can help make your wants and needs a reality. Lastly, you can look back over your notes someday to see if you have made progress. So invest in a journal, make a cup of something, and write.

FAF Midlife Reality #11: Balance: Here Today, Gone Tomorrow

When we talk about balance, we're not referring just to our crazy mixed-up lives of managing families, businesses and often aging parents. We're talking about balance—where we stand on one leg. What's more, midlife seems to be where older adults start to lose their balance. There are varying reasons for that including past inner ear infections, a predisposition to vertigo, a weakening of the core muscles, or a decline in the part of the brain that stores this function.

However, there is hope. There is solid, medical proof that if you balance on one leg regularly, you can reverse this trend. So by all means, add balancing to your day. Practice Tree Pose at the market. Stand on one leg while you are checking out at the library. Try a handstand when you try on clothes to see how they look upside-down. The better we can balance, the less likely we will stumble and suffer a devastating fall, especially in our later years. Balancing today brings a better tomorrow.

---

[21] Adrian Furnham, PhD, "Writing as Therapy," Psychology Today, August 29, 2013.

FAF Midlife Reality #12:
Companionship Feeds Our Spirit Animal

There is nothing more important than camaraderie on this road. It has inspired us to write this book to find each of you. The sense of solidarity is at the core of what it means to be human. At heart, we are pack animals. We are not meant to do this alone.

We want to encourage you to find a like-minded individual, or two, or three. Volunteer! Join up! Investigate a studio. Go into the community center. Be part of something you have a passion about. Try a movie or a book club. If your friends do not want to ride a bike, or take a walk, or practice yoga, make new ones! It's not easy, but it is doable and so very worth it. The internet has made us more isolated, not less, so you will have to get out of your house and make friends the old-fashioned way by saying hello.

The Way Home

We cannot go back and write a new beginning to our lives, but every day is a chance to make a new ending. Midlife is an opportunity to make the second half the finish we deserve. We can thrive well into our later years. Flourishing and taking care of yourself is a learned behavior. It's a choice, and just like yoga, it happens mostly on the inside.

Although we don't have all the answers, and we aren't nearly perfect, we have a plan and a path. Despite our bumps and bruises, our heartbreak, loss and pain, we firmly believe the Universe conspires for us. We want and deserve happiness, which starts with a willingness and a fearlessness to be present for it all.

If there is a God, or St. Peter, or Buddha, or Zeus, or Abraham, or Mohammed, or Archangel Gabriel, or the Tooth Fairy—if someone is there to greet us at the end of this crazy journey, and they ask us, "How was your life?" We hope you can say:

"I had one with everything."

Fearlessness comes with practice and preparation. Love, trust, hope, optimism, gratitude and generosity are all stronger than the fear that resides in our mind. Try not to let the mind dominate the conversation. Let your strong body, fearless heart, and resilient spirit help you embrace the fullest experience of life.

Aging does not mean that we have to settle for less. Time becomes more valuable, so we learn to squeeze every bit of pleasure out of every minute. It's our way of finding more in the moment.

See your life as a grand adventure, and it will be one. Let yoga be your constant light, and let the practice grow you. As you flourish on the mat, so you will in life. Make happiness your priority. Choose it. Decide on it. Affirm it, and you will thrive.

No one saves us but ourselves.
No one can and no one may.
We ourselves must walk the path.
~ **Buddha**

Om Lokah Samastah Sukhino Bhavantu
May all beings be happy and free.
May our actions cause harm to none.

Om Shanti, Shanti, Shanti
Peace, peace, peace

Abhaya
And fearlessness along the way.

We are so happy to have your company in this great adventure called life.

Lovingly,
Desiree and Michelle

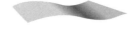

Yoga Poses:
Our Time to Thrive

Let's Practice!

It is our deepest hope that you begin to see yoga not as a way to get a pose, but as a means to get a life. We want everyone to be strong and vibrant. Yoga is our path, and it's a proven one. Try to incorporate yoga into your daily life in a way that you enjoy. Here are a few suggestions:

Dedicate a Space

Create a cozy practice space for yourself somewhere in your home. Keep your yoga mat, blanket and blocks nearby so they invite you "in." If your mat is out, you are more likely to use it. If company is coming over, suggest they practice yoga with you, too!

Make a Commitment

Make a promise to practice one or two poses and see what happens. Study how your body feels in a pose. Examine your breathing, and notice your level of mindful presence.

Find a Teacher

Find a knowledgeable teacher and attend class regularly. If you are practicing at home, going to a class even just once a week can correct your form and enhance your experience. Practice does not make perfect, but perfect practice does.

Find a Group

The energy of a class is very inspiring. Like-minded beings keep us on our way with joy and laughter. Online classes can help you learn how to sequence, and pay attention to your body.

Meditation Is Rejuvenation

Make time for a meditation of any type. Even if you sit quietly with your hot morning beverage, this is the simplest centering habit there is. This practice will leave you with more presence and peace.

"Practice and all is coming." ~ Sri K. Pattabhi Jois
To see a video tutorial of all of our yoga,
go to *www.YogaDownload.com*

Fearless After Fifty: Practical Advice Fueling Our Life

Easy and inexpensive

- Maintain your optimum weight.

- Buy local, fresh vegetables and fruits.

- Shop the perimeter of the grocery aisles.

- Avoid processed foods, and limit sugar and other known inflammatory items.

More ... money, time and focus

- Buy a juicer or high-powered blender.

- Triple your vegetable consumption with green smoothies once a day.

- Eat at farm-to-table restaurants.

- Take time to prepare high quality meals you can eat throughout your week.

All in!

- Do a fancy cleanse or food test for allergies and sensitivities.

- Join a weight loss or fitness group.

- Book an organic, vegan retreat to kick-start a new lifestyle.

- Hire a conscious chef to come to your home and teach you how to cook.

There's Always More ...

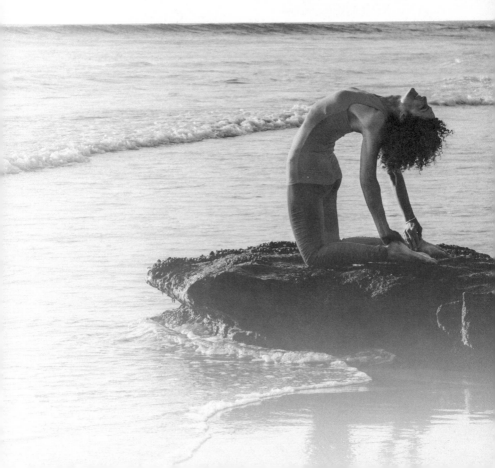

One More Thing:
FAQ About Yoga and Midlife

How is the *Fearless After Fifty* approach to yoga different than others?

It is common to feel that once a person reaches a certain age, whatever that "age" may be, the safest approach to a yoga practice is to take it easy. We were once told that the age to slow down is a puckish 40! While "gentle" yoga is sometimes necessary at any age, we believe that if you want to stay strong, you need to practice strong by using your muscles. Having a gentle and relaxed approach all the time will give you less strength, not more.

Is yoga enough to stay strong and healthy in midlife?

We wish! But sadly, no. Once we turn 50, we begin to lose muscle mass and endurance at an alarming rate. While yoga arm balances and inversions build strength, in our experience we've had to add weight work regularly since midlife. Both of us supplement our yoga practice by lifting light to medium heavy weights. Michelle also practices Pilates on a regular basis to tone her core.

Can a "flow" yoga practice build cardio endurance?

Maybe. How fast are you going? In our experience, moving with breath in a dance-like motion does not raise your heartbeat to 50% to 85% of your maximum heart rate, which is what sports experts recommend. You can use a heart rate monitor to check your performance. Both of us supplement our week with a cardio workout, either walking, running, jogging, biking, or elliptical work.

If I feel blah, should I exercise?

Depression is not a part of the normal human experience of aging. Yoga and exercise have been shown to raise our "feel good" hormones. A workout a day keeps depression away, so try to get up and get going even if you don't truly feel like it.

Can I practice yoga if my balance is not good?

We lose balance with age. Yoga reverses this process and can help us balance like a cat with nine lives! The more we practice balancing, the better we get, and the less likely we'll suffer a debilitating fall someday. Practice near a wall or holding onto a chair and never, ever give up.

Am I too inflexible for yoga?

Other falsehoods in this category include being too dirty to take a shower, and being too slow to take a walk. If you practice, it will come.

What should I look for in a yoga teacher?

Midlife yogis have special needs. We have older tendons, ligaments and muscles. Our balance is probably compromised. Our core may be weaker. We may be crazy stiff from sitting in a chair for half a century at work. It may take us longer to regain or even discover our strength and flexibility.

Look for compassion and expertise in a yoga teacher. Personally, we also appreciate someone who is near our age and in the trenches with us. That's not to say that a young teacher fresh out of her Yoga Teacher Training isn't qualified. We know some very good novice teachers who are trained in alignment, anatomy and the aging process. But that is more the exception than the rule.

My teacher tell me I'm too old for arm balances. Should I sit them out?

Balderdash and twiddle twaddle. Find a new teacher who is willing to work with you safely, patiently, and will encourage you along the way.

What is a Wisdom Warrior™ teacher?

Desiree offers a training called Wisdom Warriors where she shows yoga teachers how to carefully encourage older yogis into a more challenging practice. Those who have studied with Desiree are probably going to have a safe and centered approach to getting stronger with yoga.

What is the best yoga?

There are countless variations including Laughing Yoga and Crying Yoga, Man Yoga and Female Yoga. There is Aerial Yoga hanging from silks, and Partner Yoga hanging from a friend. We want you to do the yoga that you enjoy. If you like it, you will stick with it.

Should I try Vinyasa or Power Yoga?

We love movement! However movement doesn't always love a midlife yogi. Yoga poses don't cause nearly as much damage as moving in and out of them mindlessly. When you move, you need to pay attention. Transitions between poses are where you are likely to strain or tear something. Classes that move slowly and focus on one pose at a time are the safest overall in our experience. There is absolutely nothing wrong with enjoying a Vinyasa practice. We just ask that you stay mindful when you move, and don't zone out during class.

Should I practice heated yoga?

One of us loves it, and one of us thinks it's gross. However, we can agree that practicing in a hot room is for skilled yogis. You must be acutely aware of your body and its limitations because the heat will hide most pain until later when you realize you cannot walk.

Should I try Inversions in the middle of the room?

Midlife, when our bones are more brittle and our balance is challenged, is not the best time to learn a handstand in the middle of a room. There is some likelihood you may fall. If you feel confident upside down, please go for it. However, if you are just beginning yoga, then take your inversions to a wall where you can learn them safely. Whereas a young'un will bounce right back from toppling over, we can literally break a hip. You must weigh risk versus reward. You can reap 99.9% of the benefits of an inversion at the wall, or propped on chairs and blocks, without incurring 99.9% of the risk.

**My teacher had us do a 20-minute Shoulderstand.
Is this safe?**

Timings bring challenges and also advantages in building strength. If you set the pose up incorrectly, you will do much more potential damage than good. Always be sure your pose is aligned correctly, and have the teacher check it, before you attempt to hold it for more than a few breaths. Another good rule is that if you can no longer "work" a pose, meaning find new strength, alignment and greater relief, then it is time to come down or out of it.

Should I practice Headstand or Shoulderstand?

This is a very good question, and we unfortunately cannot answer it absolutely without seeing your practice. The "King" and "Queen" of yoga poses are the Headstand and Shoulder-stand, yet like most sovereign rulers, these two come with a certain level of risk. Both require a strong, engaged core and the strength to lift the body upwards, so the weight is not crashing into the neck and your fragile cervical spine. Many of us think we are this strong, but in actuality we are dumping into our neck. The neck is meant to support an 11-pound head, not a 175-pound body. Please learn these poses from a qualified professional. Check your neck for any signs of load bearing. And if you need to have a conscious uncoupling from these two poses, know you are not the first to go down this path.

Are there any other poses I should be wary of?

If you are an experienced, strong, longtime practitioner, there's nothing you can't do at any age. However, many of us in the West started yoga later in life. In India, a child may begin practicing yoga at age five, so they have learned to use their core and full body in poses. Those of us who start later have a significant difference in body awareness and capability. In addition to Headstand and Shoulderstand, be aware of any pose that puts pressure on your joints and ligaments. Holding Hero's Pose, *Supta Virasana*, for too long may cause a dangerous loss of blood supply to your knees. In Downward Facing Dog, use your entire hand strength and core, and don't put too much weight on the wrists. The same is true in Upward Facing Dog and Arm Balances. Be sure your shoulder blades are on your back and not rounded forward in *Chaturanga*. Be mindful of any knee or joint pain. Most importantly of all, please learn yoga from a highly qualified professional; then there is nothing you (probably) can't do.

Is Yin Yoga safe?

Lots of people love Yin, which is a gentle, restorative yoga involving long holds, often propped, without any, or minimal muscle resistance. Yet it's the muscles that keep our fragile tendons from load bearing. The benefit of Yin is that you can deepen a stretch into the fascia. The risk is that when you hang into your ligaments, the ligaments weaken over time. We know a midlife yogi who tore her hip labrum from sitting in Half Pigeon Pose for too long. Yin is not for everybody or every body; you've been warned.

How often should I practice yoga?

There is no limit to how often we can move our bodies. You can practice every day, twice a day, or less. If you do a lot of standing poses one day, you might opt for a seated practice the next, and so forth. If you feel like you are doing too much, you probably are, and the same goes for doing too little. You will know best what is right for you.

Should I try to keep up with the others in a class?

That darn ego. If our diminishing capacities don't give our self-esteem a hard enough time, along comes the competitive yoga class. To be clear, yoga is not a competition, ever, unless you are actually in the formal yoga competition held annually by USA Yoga. That does not mean that our ego takes the day off when we are in a class, though. If your ego, or mind, pipes up, thank it for sharing. Then make a qualified, adult decision about whether to keep up with a class or sit something out. The only mistake you can make is not being aware. Being conscious and careful is never a mistake.

Is it me? Why doesn't the studio feel welcoming?

You want to find a yoga community that feels inclusive and a place where everybody knows your name. If you don't feel welcomed, then try somewhere else. You want to find a group that feels good physically, and is also good company for this journey. We hope you make new a new habit of practice and new friends as well. Whatever you decide, remember, yoga is all about you. You are the yo' in yoga!

And Another...
Fifty Things to Love About Being 50

By Michelle Marchildon, The Yogi Muse[22]

While being 50 is not exactly the new 30, it isn't all bad news. In fact, I kind of like it.

Being 50 means I fail more, flail more, and generally worry about the outcome less. I take more risks and handle change because I've had plenty of it. And although there are yoga poses I won't do, and clothes I won't wear, and men I won't sleep with, there's a whole lot about being 50 that rocks.

For those who are reaching this milestone, know this for sure: It gets better. What I know now that I wish I knew then: Do not wait for an age to get this attitude.

In no particular order, here are 50 things I love about being 50:

1. Knowing who I am, and everyone else can get over it. Transparency is liberating.

2. Flirting. I've always been a flirt, but now it's ridiculous because who is going to take me seriously? Flirting is love in a wink. I flirt with everyone, from 20-somethings to octogenarians, men and women alike.

---

[22] Originally published on October 18, 2013 in the *Elephant Journal*. Reprinted with Permission.

3. I "buy" Thanksgiving. I used to think holidays weren't complete until everyone else was as miserable as I was in the kitchen. Now I buy most of it, and guess what? The world did not end.

4. The loss of the frontal lobe. Sayonara. As we age, this part of our brain deteriorates, so we say what we mean, and mean what we say. How refreshing.

5. I no longer listen to music I don't like, including anything that sounds like a car accident.

6. I no longer sleep with people I don't like, except for my husband, who I love, but not necessarily after a weekend of football, beer, brats, and chips.

7. I am vocal and clear about what I want, which took me years of self-empowerment.

8. I'm happy to have a few excellent friends. Furthermore, if I'm hurt, I move on. There's another wonderful person waiting in the future.

9. I no longer bother with cleaning the house or buying food for company. I offer whatever I have on hand and it usually seems to be enough.

10. I believe in God, and I'm clear on that. I don't pray to trees, or wiccans or anything involving sex on a rug. Not that there's anything wrong with it …. But it's not for me.

11. I try not to cause harm. I take care of other beings. And I have learned to hold my tongue and most of my opinions if they are hurtful.

12. I live simply and mostly in the present. I don't have energy or interest in the drama.

13. I tidy my house, and take care of my body, and I realize that divinity has been inside all along (thank you, B.K.S. Iyengar).

14. I love my yoga practice, which is new for me. Twenty years ago I wanted to do every pose, perfectly. These days I am grateful to touch my toes.

15. Yet there are some poses that I no longer practice, such as the transition from Handstand to *Chaturanga*. We had a messy break-up involving broken toes, but I'm over it now.

16. Gratitude in general. Big love to gratitude. I am moved to tears by the little things.

17. I'm still here. Every. Damn. Day. Fifty is old, but the alternative is worse.

18. I live with minimal regrets, seeing the humanity and compassion of it all.

19. I say I'm sorry. This was never hard for me, but now after 50, it is somehow even easier. Humans are clumsy and cause harm, so we need to fix it when we stumble.

20. But I don't apologize for being me. I'm done with that. If others feel less than or insecure, that is their problem and they can own it.

21. I do small kindnesses for complete strangers. It's a total rush.

22. And I do big kindnesses for my friends.

23. I don't take much seriously or personally. I have no idea why I didn't understand this earlier.

24. I laugh, especially at myself. When I die, I hope it's from having a heart attack while laughing.

25. I am much more generous. If you can't take it with you, then give more of it away.

26. I do not care as much about how I look in jeans. And I wear a bikini. Nothing looks as good as confidence. Of course, my kids won't be seen with me in public.

27. I am less concerned with the scale and the number. I have been a size 0, a size 12, and a size 42 in Paris. What matters is if you feel healthy.

28. After 50 years of fighting it, I now love my belly. I have two wonderful children and I wouldn't trade them for six-pack abs.

29. However, I am fighting the good fight for my face. A little maintenance goes a long way.

30. I'm not ashamed to admit that I love my car. I freaking love my car! If you think that's materialistic, or spiritually bankrupt, then obviously you do not have the same car.

31. My family matters. Evenings and weekends are the most lucrative times to teach yoga, but I won't do it until my youngest goes to college.

32. I waited a very long time to put myself first. Now it's my turn to write, to travel, to do whatever.

33. Realizing that nothing changes. We know more now. So when I find out about disloyalty and other human flaws, I know it was a gift to have it revealed.

34. I'm over the answers. I'm okay with "I don't know." And I'm excited to learn anew.

35. I'm good with failure. I can fail all day long. I can fall out of handstand, I can flail in a yoga pose, and I can even write a terrible blog because I know there's another chance to get it right.

36. I no longer dress to look young. I'm happy with looking 50, whatever that means.

37. I like my tribe. Finding like-minded people has been the best part of the journey.

38. I've forgiven almost everyone who has done shit to me, and there were a lot. I am working on the others, but in truth, I feel there are some malicious acts that should not be forgiven, such as harming your children or defenseless animals.

39. However, I never carry a grudge. Why bother? I'd rather carry a Louis Vuitton.

40. I'm getting used to change. I'm not in control, and it's a relief. The Universe is in control.

41. Instead of worrying, I clean. Clean what you can, and the Universe will take care of the rest.

42. I am a conscious eater. I am mostly a vegetarian who eats a little bit of free-range chicken, and occasionally humanely-raised bacon. I don't feel that makes me a bad person.

43. I shop for karma. Diet is not the only way to change the world. A fabric bag with leather trim is almost vegan, and almost is better than not at all.

44. I am teaching slower yoga and a more refined movement, which seems to be limiting my appeal. I'm fine with working my way down the ladder because it feels right for me now.

45. I'd rather be authentic than popular. I've been both, and I know which helps me sleep at night.

46. I've learned a thing or two. I would never, ever, go back to my 20s.

47. I'm a strong, capable, competent woman, and I'm okay if some people spell that B-I-T-C-H.

48. I appreciate my weaknesses, because they are often my strengths.

49. I say "Thank you," instead of "F@$k you." It might be my greatest accomplishment coming from New York.

50. Lastly, I know my dharma. I am better, stronger and wiser. Decisions come easier. Life is lighter. I am happier. It's taken me 50 years and all I can say is it is better late, than never.

Whoever you are, wherever you are, enjoy your later years. It is much better than the alternative.

We Can't Stop!
Recipes from the
Fearless Foodie cookbook

*Let food be thy medicine
and medicine be thy food.*
~ Hippocrates

Desiree loves to cook, which also makes her the perfect houseguest. Here is a sample taken from the *Fearless Foodie* cookbook, which she wrote with her daughter, Jessica Gouthro.

These recipes rely on healthy, natural and organic foods, limiting, if not completely avoiding, the most well-known inflammatory substances such as dairy, wheat, gluten and sugar.

Bon appetit!

Classic Green Smoothie (serves 2)

Incorporating more greens, fruits and vegetables into our diet gives us energy galore and a power-packed drink of nutrients. Ginger and turmeric increase the anti-inflammatory properties.

1 T. fresh ginger
1 T. fresh turmeric (optional)

2 large kale leaves

2 large chard leaves

2 sprigs parsley

½ cup chopped cucumber

2 large leaves lettuce

1 cup spinach

1 medium apple

½ avocado

1 cup water, or use almond or coconut milk if you want a richer drink

Wash and roughly chop veggies. Blend ingredients together preferably in a high-speed blender. Depending on how sweet you want it to be, you can add frozen fruit (blueberries, bananas, mango, pineapple, etc.). You can also add cacao nibs, unsweetened shredded coconut, in addition to other superfoods or protein supplements such as collagen powder.

Quinoa Walnut Falafels (6 servings, about 3 per serving, or 20 small patties)

A healthy update to falafel balls that you can enjoy alone or add to a salad. These pack a powerful protein punch from the quinoa.

1½ cups cooked quinoa

1 celery stalk

½ large onion

2 garlic cloves
1 shredded carrot
1 cup raw walnuts
1 cup fresh parsley
½ cup fresh basil
1 t. dried thyme
1½ cups Coconut Aminos, Tamari, or any gluten-free seasoning sauce
Salt and pepper to taste

Preheat oven to 400 degrees. Lightly grease a baking sheet with coconut oil or spray.

Sauté the celery, onion, garlic, carrot mixture.

Stir in the cooked quinoa to warm it up.

Put the walnuts, herbs and coconut aminos in a food processor. Combine. Then add the celery/onion sauté after it cools.

Add salt and pepper to taste.

Blend until it is soft enough to form patties.

Use hands to scoop out a portion and roll it up into a golf ball size. Smoosh it out a bit on the baking sheet to make it look like a small burger.

Bake for approximately 20 minutes or until browned.

Serve wrapped in a leaf of lettuce with sliced tomatoes and Tahini Sauce.

Tahini Sauce (Yummy Sauce)

Use this on burgers, fish, chicken, or anything that needs a little boost in flavor.

¼ cup miso
½ cup tahini
Juice of 1 lemon (or to taste)
½ cup water

Blend all ingredients together and adjust taste to your preference. You can add Coconut Aminos or tamari sauce to taste and thin with water to desired consistency.

Herbed Turkey Burgers (serves 8)

A healthy and tasteful substitute for the classic burger. Try serving these wrapped in lettuce rather than a bun. You get a nice added crunch without any additional calories.

2 lb. ground turkey
1 red onion, minced
4 garlic cloves, minced
Egg, optional
1 t. sea salt
1 t. black pepper
½ cup chopped parsley
1 T. rosemary
1 T. sage
2 t. thyme

Sauté onions and garlic in coconut oil. Once they are cool, mix them into the turkey by hand and add all of the seasonings. Cook on a hot grill or sauté in a pan for 5 minutes each side.

You may also add an egg to the mixture to keep it extra moist. Delicious served with mustard!

Banana Walnut Bread (yield 1 gluten-free loaf)

Our favorite decadent treat. While it is gluten-free, and guilt-free, we can't guarantee that it is calorie-free. It works well for special occasions; people always ask for this recipe.

Wet ingredients:
10 dried dates, pitted
2 ripe bananas
$^1/_3$ cup maple syrup
¼ cup virgin coconut oil, melted
2 T. lemon juice
1 t. vanilla extract

Dry ingredients:
1 cup chickpea flour
1 cup almond meal
¼ cup tapioca flour
1 T. baking powder
1 t. baking soda
½ t. ground cinnamon
½ t. sea salt

Preheat oven to 350 degrees and lightly grease 8 x 11 baking dish.

Place dates in large bowl and cover with boiling water to soften.

Drain well, then add bananas and mash both together so that chunks remain.

Add maple syrup, melted oil, lemon juice and vanilla.

Whisk to combine.

In separate bowl, whisk together dry ingredients. Add to bowl with banana mixture and bake for 30 minutes or until toothpick inserted in center comes out clean. Remove from oven, place on rack and cool completely before slicing.

About the Authors

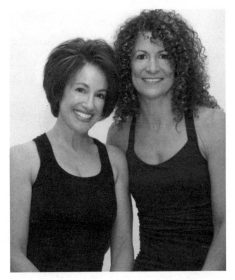

Desiree Rumbaugh is an international yoga teacher with an unquenchable enthusiasm for life, love and healing. Desiree travels the world full-time sharing her compassion and her joy with others interested in the transformational power of yoga. She blends playful humor with an authentic inquiry into the nature of *being* in order to bring the ancient teachings of wisdom into modern life.

With longtime studies in Iyengar and Anusara yoga, she is an E-500 RYT and brings 30 years of experience to her ever-evolving style. She is the creator of the *Yoga to the Rescue* DVD series for back, neck and shoulder pain. You can find her videos online with Gaia, Yoginit, Tintyoga and YogaDownload. She co-wrote the *Fearless Foodie* cookbook with her daughter, Jessica Gouthro. Desiree is a regular contributor to *Yoga Journal*, having also appeared on its cover.

Her charitable work includes supporting the Art of Yoga Project serving teenage girls in the juvenile justice system. You can find her at *www.DesireeRumbaugh.com*. She lives with her husband, Andrew Rivin, in Southern California.

Michelle Berman Marchildon is The Yogi Muse. She's an award-winning journalist, author and columnist. You can find her writings in *Yoga Journal, Yoga International, Mantra Yoga and Health, Origin Magazine, Elephant Journal,* and *Sports Illustrated.* She is an alumni of the Columbia University Graduate School of Journalism.

Her other books include, *Finding More on the Mat: How I Grew Better, Wiser and Stronger through Yoga* (Hohm Press, 2015), and *Theme Weaver: Connect the Power of Inspiration to Teaching Yoga* (Wildhorse Ventures, 2014.) She has been practicing yoga regularly since 1995 and is an E-RYT 500 certified teacher. Michelle supports the rights and sanctuaries of animals worldwide.

You can find her blog and website at *www.YogiMuse.com*. She has videos on *www.YogaDownload.com*. She teaches and resides in Denver, Colorado.

About the Photographers

- Cover Photograph: David Martinez of David Martinez Studio. Photograph taken when Desiree was just a youthful 48, looking forward to being fearless in her fifties.

- Back Cover, photos of Desiree and Michelle: Kimberly Benfield, K. Benfield Photography.

- Desiree on a rock, Mario Covic Photography

- Desiree with Groups: Karen Church Photography

Index